HEALTH AND HUMAN DEVELOPMENT

MEXICO

HEALTH AND AGING

HEALTH AND HUMAN DEVELOPMENT

JOAV MERRICK - SERIES EDITOR

NATIONAL INSTITUTE OF CHILD HEALTH
AND HUMAN DEVELOPMENT,
MINISTRY OF SOCIAL AFFAIRS, JERUSALEM

Mexico: Health and Aging
Supa Pengpid, Karl Peltzer and Joav Merrick (Editors)
2020. ISBN: 978-1-53617-950-7 (Softcover)
2020. ISBN: 978-1-53617-951-4 (eBook)

Clinical Oncology: An Encompassing Overview
Joav Merrick, Ariel Tenenbaum, Victoria Rico and Carlo DeAngelis (Editors)
2020. ISBN: 978-1-53617-933-0 (Hardcover)
2020. ISBN. 978-1-53617-934-7 (eBook)

Pain: Perspectives on Acute and Chronic Pain
Patricia Schofield, Ariel Tenenbaum, Joav Merrick (Editors)
2020: ISBN: 978-1-53617-748-0 (Hardcover)
2020: ISBN: 978-1-53617-749-7 (eBook)

Animal-Assisted Interventions for Health and Human Service Professionals
Carlie J. Driscoll
2020. ISBN: 978-1-53617-433-5 (Hardcover)
2020. ISBN: 978-1-53617-434-2 (eBook)

Cancer Management in Latin America II: Melanoma to Cost-Effectiveness
Maurício F Silva, Gustavo Nader Marta, Luis CM Antunes, Fiona Lim, Bo Angela Wan, Beatriz Amendola, Joav Merrick (Editors)
2020. ISBN: 978-1-53616-735-1 (Hardcover)
2020. ISBN: 978-1-53616-736-8 (eBook)

Cancer Management in Latin America I: Nasopharyngeal to Renal Cancer
Maurício F Silva, Gustavo Nader Marta, Luis CM Antunes, Fiona Lim, Bo Angela Wan, Beatriz Amendola, Joav Merrick (Editors)
2020. ISBN: 978-1-53616-733-7 (Hardcover)
2020. ISBN: 978-1-53616-734-4 (eBook)

Clinical Art Psychotherapy with War Veterans
Alexander Kopytin and Alexey Lebedev
2018. ISBN: 978-1-53612-975-5 (Softcover)
2017. ISBN: 978-1-53612-976-2 (eBook)

Cancer and Exercise
Leila Malek, Fiona Lim, Bo Angela Wan, Patrick L Diaz, Edward Chow, Joav Merrick (Editors)
2018. ISBN: 978-1-53612-747-8 (Hardcover)
2018. ISBN: 978-1-53612-748-5 (eBook)

Brennan Healing Science: An Integrative Approach to Therapeutic Intervention
Nina Koren, Muriel Moreno and Joav Merrick (Editors)
2018. ISBN: 978-1-53612-825-3 (Hardcover)
2018. ISBN: 978-1-53612-826-0 (eBook)

Alternative Medicine Research Yearbook 2017
Joav Merrick (Editor)
2018. ISBN: 978-1-53613-726-2 (Hardcover)
2018. ISBN: 978-1-53613-727-9 (eBook)

Psychosocial Needs: Success in Life and Career Planning
Daniel TL Shek, Janet TY Leung, Tak Y Lee and Joav Merrick (Editors)
2017. ISBN: 978-1-53611-951-0 (Hardcover)
2017. ISBN: 978-1-53611-971-8 (eBook)

Cannabis: Medical Aspects
Blair Henry, Arnav Agarwal, Edward Chow, Hatim A Omar, and Joav Merrick (Editors)
2017. ISBN: 978-1-53610-510-0 (Hardcover)
2017. ISBN: 978-1-53610-522-3 (eBook)

Palliative Care: Oncology Experience from Hong Kong
Louisa Cheuk-Yu Lui, Kam-Hung Wong, Rebecca Yeung, Joav Merrick (Editors)
2017. ISBN: 978-1-53612-397-5 (Softcover)
2017. ISBN: 978-1-53612-430-9 (eBook)

Palliative Care: Psychosocial and Ethical Considerations
Blair Henry, Arnav Agarwal, Edward Chow, and Joav Merrick (Editors)
2017. ISBN: 978-1-53610-607-7 (Hardcover)
2017. ISBN: 978-1-53610-611-4 (eBook)

Oncology: The Promising Future of Biomarkers
Anthony Furfari, George S Charames, Rachel McDonald, Leigha Rowbottom, Azar Azad, Stephanie Chan, Bo Angela Wan, Ronald Chow, Carlo DeAngelis, Pearl Zaki, Edward Chow and Joav Merrick (Editors)
2017. ISBN: 978-1-53610-608-4 (Hardcover)
2017. ISBN: 978-1-53610-610-7 (eBook)

Public Health Yearbook 2016
Joav Merrick (Editor)
2017. ISBN: 978-1-53610-947-4 (Hardcover)
2017. ISBN: 978-1-53610-956-6 (eBook)

Alternative Medicine Research Yearbook 2016
Joav Merrick (Editor)
2017. ISBN: 978-1-53610-972-6 (Hardcover)
2017. ISBN: 978-1-53611-000-5 (eBook)

Pain Management Yearbook 2016
Joav Merrick (Editor)
2017. ISBN: 978-1-53610-949-8 (Hardcover)
2017. ISBN: 978-1-53610-959-7 (eBook)

Medical Cannabis: Clinical Practice
Shannon O'Hearn, Alexia Blake, Bo Angela Wan, Stephanie Chan, Edward Chow and Joav Merrick (Editors)
2017. ISBN: 978-1-53611-907-7 (Softcover)
2017. ISBN: 978-1-53611-927-5 (eBook)

Cancer: Treatment, Decision Making and Quality of Life
Breanne Lechner, Ronald Chow, Natalie Pulenzas, Marko Popovic, Na Zhang, Xiaojing Zhang, Edward Chow, and Joav Merrick (Editors)
2016. ISBN: 978-1-63483-863-4 (Hardcover)
2015. ISBN: 978-1-63483-882-5 (eBook)

Cancer: Bone Metastases, CNS Metastases and Pathological Fractures
Breanne Lechner, Ronald Chow, Natalie Pulenzas, Marko Popovic, Na Zhang, Xiaojing Zhang, Edward Chow, and Joav Merrick (Editors)
2016. ISBN: 978-1-63483-949-5 (Hardcover)
2015. ISBN: 978-1-63483-960-0 (eBook)

Cancer: Spinal Cord, Lung, Breast, Cervical, Prostate, Head and Neck Cancer
Breanne Lechner, Ronald Chow, Natalie Pulenzas, Marko Popovic, Na Zhang, Xiaojing Zhang, Edward Chow and Joav Merrick (Editors)
2016. ISBN: 978-1-63483-904-4 (Hardcover)
2015. ISBN: 978-1-63483-911-2 (eBook)

Cancer: Survival, Quality of Life and Ethical Implications
Breanne Lechner, Ronald Chow, Natalie Pulenzas, Marko Popovic, Na Zhang, Xiaojing Zhang, Edward Chow and Joav Merrick (Editors)
2016. ISBN: 978-1-63483-905-1 (Hardcover)
2015. ISBN: 978-1-63483-912-9 (eBook)

Cancer: Pain and Symptom Management
Breanne Lechner, Ronald Chow, Natalie Pulenzas, Marko Popovic, Na Zhang, Xiaojing Zhang, Edward Chow, and Joav Merrick (Editors)
2016. ISBN: 978-1-63483-905-1 (Hardcover)
2015. ISBN: 978-1-63483-881-8 (eBook)

Alternative Medicine Research Yearbook 2015
Joav Merrick (Editor)
2016. ISBN: 978-1-63484-511-3 (Hardcover)
2016. ISBN: 978-1-63484-542-7 (eBook)

Public Health Yearbook 2015
Joav Merrick (Editor)
2016. ISBN: 978-1-63484-511-3 (Hardcover)
2016. ISBN: 978-1-63484-546-5 (eBook)

Quality, Mobility and Globalization in the Higher Education System: A Comparative Look at the Challenges of Academic Teaching
Nitza Davidovitch, Zehavit Gross, Yuri Ribakov, and Anna Slobodianiuk (Editors)
2016. ISBN: 978-1-63484-986-9 (Hardcover)
2016. ISBN: 978-1-63485-012-4 (eBook)

Alternative Medicine Research Yearbook 2014
Joav Merrick (Editor)
2015. ISBN: 978-1-63482-161-2 (Hardcover)
2015. ISBN: 978-1-63482-205-3 (eBook)

Pain Management Yearbook 2014
Joav Merrick (Editor)
2015. ISBN: 978-1-63482-164-3 (Hardcover)
2015. ISBN: 978-1-63482-208-4 (eBook)

Public Health Yearbook 2014
Joav Merrick (Editor)
2015. ISBN: 978-1-63482-165-0 (Hardcover)
2015. ISBN: 978-1-63482-209-1 (eBook)

Forensic Psychiatry: A Public Health Perspective
Leo Sher and Joav Merrick (Editors)
2015. ISBN: 978-1-63483-339-4 (Hardcover)
2015. ISBN: 978-1-63483-346-2 (eBook)

Leadership and Service Learning Education: Holistic Development for Chinese University Students
Daniel TL Shek, Florence KY Wu and Joav Merrick (Editors)
2015. ISBN: 978-1-63483-340-0 (Hardcover)
2015. ISBN: 978-1-63483-347-9 (eBook)

Mental and Holistic Health: Some International Perspectives
Joseph L Calles Jr, Donald E Greydanus, and Joav Merrick (Editors)
2015. ISBN: 978-1-63483-589-3 (Hardcover)
2015. ISBN: 978-1-63483-608-1 (eBook)

India: Health and Human Development Aspects
Joav Merrick (Editor)
2014. ISBN: 978-1-62948-784-7 (Hardcover)
2014. ISBN: 978-1-62948-794-6 (eBook)

Alternative Medicine Research Yearbook 2013
Joav Merrick (Editor)
2014. ISBN: 978-1-63321-094-3 (Hardcover)
2014. ISBN: 978-1-63321-144-5 (eBook)

Health Consequences of Human Central Obesity
Kaushik Bose and Raja Chakraborty (Editors)
2014. ISBN: 978-1-63321-152-0 (Hardcover)
2014. ISBN: 978-1-63321-181-0 (eBook)

Public Health: Improving Health via Inter-Professional Collaborations
Rosemary M Caron and Joav Merrick (Editors)
2014. ISBN: 978-1-63321-569-6 (Hardcover)
2014. ISBN: 978-1-63321-594-8 (eBook)

Public Health Yearbook 2013
Joav Merrick (Editor)
2014. ISBN: 978-1-63321-095-0 (Hardcover)
2014. ISBN: 978-1-63321-097-4 (eBook)

Textbook on Evidence-Based Holistic Mind-Body Medicine: Holistic Practice of Traditional Hippocratic Medicine
Søren Ventegodt and Joav Merrick
2013. ISBN: 978-1-62257-105-5 (Hardcover)
2012. ISBN: 978-1-62257-174-1 (eBook)

Textbook on Evidence-Based Holistic Mind-Body Medicine: Sexology and Traditional Hippocratic Medicine
Søren Ventegodt and Joav Merrick
2013. ISBN: 978-1-62257-130-7 (Hardcover)
2012. ISBN: 978-1-62257-176-5 (eBook)

Health and Happiness from Meaningful Work: Research in Quality of Working Life
Søren Ventegodt and Joav Merrick (Editors)
2013. ISBN: 978-1-60692-820-2 (Hardcover)
2009. ISBN: 978-1-61324-981-9 (eBook)

Textbook on Evidence-Based Holistic Mind-Body Medicine: Healing the Mind in Traditional Hippocratic Medicine
Søren Ventegodt and Joav Merrick
2013. ISBN: 978-1-62257-112-3 (Hardcover)
2012. ISBN: 978-1-62257-175-8 (eBook)

Conceptualizing Behavior in Health and Social Research: A Practical Guide to Data Analysis
Said Shahtahmasebi and Damon Berridge
2013. ISBN: 978-1-60876-383-2 (Hardcover)
2013. ISBN: 978-1-53611-212-2 (eBook)

Adolescence and Sports
Dilip R Patel, Donald E Greydanus, Hatim Omar and Joav Merrick (Editors)
2013. ISBN: 978-1-60876-702-1 (Hardcover)
2010. ISBN: 978-1-61761-483-5 (eBook)

Pediatric and Adolescent Sexuality and Gynecology: Principles for the Primary Care Clinician
Hatim A Omar, Donald E Greydanus, Artemis K. Tsitsika, Dilip R. Patel and Joav Merrick (Editors)
2013. ISBN: 978-1-60876-735-9 (Softcover)

Human Development: Biology from a Holistic Point of View
Søren Ventegodt, Tyge Dahl Hermansen and Joav Merrick
2013. ISBN: 978-1-61470-441-6 (Hardcover)
2011. ISBN: 978-1-61470-541-3 (eBook)

Building Community Capacity: Case Examples from Around the World
Rosemary M Caron and Joav Merrick (Editors)
2013. ISBN: 978-1-62417-175-8 (Hardcover)
2013. ISBN: 978-1-62417-176-5 (eBook)

Managed Care in a Public Setting
Richard Evan Steele
2013. ISBN: 978-1-62417-970-9 (Softcover)
2013. ISBN: 978-1-62417-863-4 (eBook)

Bullying: A Public Health Concern
Jorge C Srabstein and Joav Merrick (Editors)
2013. ISBN: 978-1-62618-564-7 (Hardcover)
2013. ISBN: 978-1-62618-588-3 (eBook)

Bedouin Health: Perspectives from Israel
Joav Merrick, Alean Al-Krenami and Salman Elbedour (Editors)
2013. ISBN: 978-1-62948-271-2 (Hardcover)
2013: ISBN: 978-1-62948-274-3 (eBook)

Health Promotion: Community Singing as a Vehicle to Promote Health
Jing Sun, Nicholas Buys and Joav Merrick (Editors)
2013. ISBN: 978-1-62618-908-9 (Hardcover)
2013: ISBN: 978-1-62808-006-3 (eBook)

Public Health Yearbook 2012
Joav Merrick (Editor)
2013. ISBN: 978-1-62808-078-0 (Hardcover)
2013: ISBN: 978-1-62808-079-7 (eBook)

Alternative Medicine Research Yearbook 2012
Joav Merrick (Editor)
2013. ISBN: 978-1-62808-080-3 (Hardcover)
2013: ISBN: 978-1-62808-079-7 (eBook)

Advanced Cancer: Managing Symptoms and Quality of Life
Natalie Pulenzas, Breanne Lechner, Nemica Thavarajah, Edward Chow, and Joav Merrick (Editors)
2013. ISBN: 978-1-62808-239-5 (Hardcover)
2013: ISBN: 978-1-62808-267-8 (eBook)

Treatment and Recovery of Eating Disorders
Daniel Stein and Yael Latzer (Editors)
2013. ISBN: 978-1-62808-248-7 (Softcover)

Health Promotion: Strengthening Positive Health and Preventing Disease
Jing Sun, Nicholas Buys and Joav Merrick (Editors)
2013. ISBN: 978-1-62257-870-2 (Hardcover)
2013: ISBN: 978-1-62808-621-8 (eBook)

Pain Management Yearbook 2011
Joav Merrick (Editor)
2013. ISBN: 978-1-62808-970-7 (Hardcover)
2013: ISBN: 978-1-62808-971-4 (eBook)

Pain Management Yearbook 2012
Joav Merrick (Editor)
2013. ISBN: 978-1-62808-973-8 (Hardcover)
2013: ISBN: 978-1-62808-974-5 (eBook)

Suicide from a Public Health Perspective
Said Shahtahmasebi and Joav Merrick
2013. ISBN: 978-1-62948-536-2 (Hardcover)
2014: ISBN: 978-1-62948-537-9 (eBook)

Food, Nutrition and Eating Behavior
Joav Merrick and Sigal Israeli (Editors)
2013. ISBN: 978-1-62948-233-0 (Hardcover)
2013: ISBN: 978-1-62948-234-7 (eBook)

Public Health Concern: Smoking, Alcohol and Substance Use
Joav Merrick and Ariel Tenenbaum (Editors)
2013. ISBN: 978-1-62948-424-2 (Hardcover)
2013. ISBN: 978-1-62948-430-3 (eBook)

Mental Health from an International Perspective
Joav Merrick, Shoshana Aspler and Mohammed Morad (Editors)
2013. ISBN: 978-1-62948-519-5 (Hardcover)
2013. ISBN: 978-1-62948-520-1 (eBook)

Adolescence and Chronic Illness. A Public Health Concern
Hatim Omar, Donald E Greydanus, Dilip R Patel and Joav Merrick (Editors)
2012. ISBN: 978-1-60876-628-4 (Hardcover)
2010. ISBN: 978-1-61761-482-8 (eBook)

Child and Adolescent Health Yearbook 2009
Joav Merrick (Editor)
2012. ISBN: 978-1-61668-913-1 (Hardcover)
2012. ISBN: 978-1-62257-095-9 (eBook)

Child and Adolescent Health Yearbook 2010
Joav Merrick (Editor)
2012. ISBN: 978-1-61209-788-6 (Hardcover)
2012. ISBN: 978-1-62417-046-1 (eBook)

Child Health and Human Development Yearbook 2010
Joav Merrick (Editor)
2012. ISBN: 978-1-61209-789-3 (Hardcover)
2012. ISBN: 978-1-62081-721-6 (eBook)

Public Health Yearbook 2010
Joav Merrick (Editor)
2012. ISBN: 978-1-61209-971-2 (Hardcover)
2012. ISBN: 978-1-62417-863-4 (eBook)

Health Risk Communication
Marijke Lemal and Joav Merrick (Editors)
2012. ISBN: 978-1-62257-544-2 (Hardcover)
2012. ISBN: 978-1-62257-552-7 (eBook)

Alternative Medicine Yearbook 2010
Joav Merrick (Editor)
2012. ISBN: 978-1-62100-132-4 (Hardcover)
2011. ISBN: 978-1-62100-210-9 (eBook)

The Astonishing Brain and Holistic Consciousness: Neuroscience and Vedanta Perspectives
Vinod D Deshmukh
2012. ISBN: 978-1-61324-295-7 (Hardcover)
2012. ISBN: 978-1-62808-677-5 (eBook)

Translational Research for Primary Healthcare
Erica Bell, Gert P Westert and Joav Merrick (Editors)
2012. ISBN: 978-1-61324-647-4 (Hardcover)
2012. ISBN: 978-1-62417-409-4 (eBook)

Building Community Capacity: Minority and Immigrant Populations
Rosemary M Caron and Joav Merrick (Editors)
2012. ISBN: 978-1-62081-022-4 (Hardcover)
2012. ISBN: 978-1-62081-032-3 (eBook)

Applied Public Health: Examining Multifaceted Social or Ecological Problems and Child Maltreatment
John R Lutzker and Joav Merrick (Editors)
2012. ISBN: 978-1-62081-356-0 (Hardcover)
2012. ISBN: 978-1-62081-388-1 (eBook)

Our Search for Meaning in Life: Quality of Life Philosophy
Søren Ventegodt and Joav Merrick
2012. ISBN: 978-1-61470-494-2 (Hardcover)
2011. ISBN: 978-1-61470-519-2 (eBook)

Randomized Clinical Trials and Placebo: Can You Trust the Drugs are Working and Safe?
Søren Ventegodt and Joav Merrick
2012. ISBN: 978-1-61470-067-8 (Hardcover)
2011. ISBN: 978-1-61470-151-4 (eBook)

Treatment and Recovery of Eating Disorders
Daniel Stein and Yael Latzer (Editors)
2012. ISBN: 978-1-61470-259-7 (Hardcover)
2012. ISBN: 978-1-61470-418-8 (eBook)

Human Immunodeficiency Virus (HIV) Research: Social Science Aspects
Hugh Klein and Joav Merrick (Editors)
2012. ISBN: 978-1-62081-293-8 (Hardcover)
2012. ISBN: 978-1-62081-346-1 (eBook)

AIDS and Tuberculosis: Public Health Aspects
Daniel Chemtob and Joav Merrick (Editors)
2012. ISBN: 978-1-62081-382-9 (Softcover)
2012. ISBN: 978-1-62081-406-2 (eBook)

Public Health Yearbook 2011
Joav Merrick (Editor)
2012. ISBN: 978-1-62081-433-8 (Hardcover)
2012. ISBN: 978-1-62081-434-5 (eBook)

Alternative Medicine Research Yearbook 2011
Joav Merrick (Editor)
2012. ISBN: 978-1-62081-476-5 (Hardcover)
2012. ISBN: 978-1-62081-477-2 (eBook)

Building Community Capacity: Skills and Principles
Rosemary M Caron and Joav Merrick (Editors)
2012. ISBN: 978-1-61209-331-4 (Hardcover)
2012. ISBN: 978-1-62257-238-0 (eBook)

Textbook on Evidence-Based Holistic Mind-Body Medicine: Basic Principles of Healing in Traditional Hippocratic Medicine
Søren Ventegodt and Joav Merrick
2012. ISBN: 978-1-62257-094-2 (Hardcover)
2012. ISBN: 978-1-62257-172-7 (eBook)

Textbook on Evidence-Based Holistic Mind-Body Medicine: Basic Philosophy and Ethics of Traditional Hippocratic Medicine
Søren Ventegodt and Joav Merrick
2012. ISBN: 978-1-62257-052-2 (Hardcover)
2013. ISBN: 978-1-62257-707-1 (eBook)

Textbook on Evidence-Based Holistic Mind-Body Medicine: Research, Philosophy, Economy and Politics of Traditional Hippocratic Medicine
Søren Ventegodt and Joav Merrick
2012. ISBN: 978-1-62257-140-6 (Hardcover)
2012. ISBN: 978-1-62257-171-0 (eBook)

Behavioral Pediatrics, 3rd Edition
Donald E Greydanus, Dilip R Patel, Helen D Pratt and Joseph L Calles, Jr (Editors)
2011. ISBN: 978-1-60692-702-1 (Hardcover)
2009. ISBN: 978-1-60876-630-7 (eBook)

Rural Child Health: International Aspects
Erica Bell and Joav Merrick (Editors)
2011. ISBN: 978-1-60876-357-3 (Hardcover)
2011. ISBN: 978-1-61324-005-2 (eBook)

International Aspects of Child Abuse and Neglect
Howard Dubowitz and Joav Merrick (Editors)
2011. ISBN: 978-1-60876-703-8 (Hardcover)
2010. ISBN: 978-1-61122-049-0 (Softcover)
2010. ISBN: 978-1-61122-403-0 (eBook)

Environment, Mood Disorders and Suicide
Teodor T Postolache and Joav Merrick (Editors)
2011. ISBN: 978-1-61668-505-8 (Hardcover)
2011. ISBN: 978-1-62618-340-7 (eBook)

Positive Youth Development: Evaluation and Future Directions in a Chinese Context
Daniel TL Shek, Hing Keung Ma and Joav Merrick (Editors)
2011. ISBN: 978-1-60876-830-1 (Hardcover)
2011. ISBN: 978-1-62100-175-1 (Softcover)
2010. ISBN: 978-1-61209-091-7 (eBook)

Understanding Eating Disorders: Integrating Culture, Psychology and Biology
Yael Latzer, Joav Merrick and Daniel Stein (Editors)
2011. ISBN: 978-1-61728-298-0 (Hardcover)
2011. ISBN: 978-1-61470-976-3 (Softcover)
2011. ISBN: 978-1-61942-054-0 (eBook)

Advanced Cancer Pain and Quality of Life
Edward Chow and Joav Merrick (Editors)
2011. ISBN: 978-1-61668-207-1 (Hardcover)
2010. ISBN: 978-1-61668-400-6 (eBook)

Positive Youth Development: Implementation of a Youth Program in a Chinese Context
Daniel TL Shek, Hing Keung Ma and Joav Merrick (Editors)
2011. ISBN: 978-1-61668-230-9

Social and Cultural Psychiatry Experience from the Caribbean Region
Hari D Maharajh and Joav Merrick (Editors)
2011. ISBN: 978-1-61668-506-5 (Hardcover)
2010. ISBN: 978-1-61728-088-7 (eBook)

Narratives and Meanings of Migration
Julia Mirsky
2011. ISBN: 978-1-61761-103-2 (Hardcover)
2010. ISBN: 978-1-61761-519-1 (eBook)

Self-Management and the Health Care Consumer
Peter William Harvey
2011. ISBN: 978-1-61761-796-6 (Hardcover)
2011. ISBN: 978-1-61122-214-2 (eBook)

Sexology from a Holistic Point of View
Soren Ventegodt and Joav Merrick
2011. ISBN: 978-1-61761-859-8 (Hardcover)
2011. ISBN: 978-1-61122-262-3 (eBook)

Principles of Holistic Psychiatry: A Textbook on Holistic Medicine for Mental Disorders
Soren Ventegodt and Joav Merrick
2011. ISBN: 978-1-61761-940-3 (Hardcover)
2011. ISBN: 978-1-61122-263-0 (eBook)

Clinical Aspects of Psychopharmacology in Childhood and Adolescence
Donald E Greydanus, Joseph L Calles, Jr, Dilip P Patel, Ahsan Nazeer and Joav Merrick (Editors)
2011. ISBN: 978-1-61122-135-0 (Hardcover)
2011. ISBN: 978-1-61122-715-4 (eBook)

Climate Change and Rural Child Health
Erica Bell, Bastian M Seidel and Joav Merrick (Editors)
2011. ISBN: 978-1-61122-640-9 (Hardcover)
2011. ISBN: 978-1-61209-014-6 (eBook)

Rural Medical Education: Practical Strategies
Erica Bell, Craig Zimitat and Joav Merrick (Editors)
2011. ISBN: 978-1-61122-649-2 (Hardcover)
2011. ISBN: 978-1-61209-476-2 (eBook)

Advances in Environmental Health Effects of Toxigenic Mold and Mycotoxins
Ebere Cyril Anyanwu
2011. ISBN: 978-1-60741-953-2
2011. ISBN: 978-1-53611-209-2

Public Health Yearbook 2009
Joav Merrick (Editor)
2011. ISBN: 978-1-61668-911-7 (Hardcover)
2011. ISBN: 978-1-62417-365-3 (eBook)

Child Health and Human Development Yearbook 2009
Joav Merrick (Editor)
2011. ISBN: 978-1-61668-912-4

Alternative Medicine Yearbook 2009
Joav Merrick (Editor)
2011. ISBN: 978-1-61668-910-0 (Hardcover)
2011. ISBN: 978-1-62081-710-0 (eBook)

The Dance of Sleeping and Eating among Adolescents: Normal and Pathological Perspectives
Yael Latzer and Orna Tzischinsky (Editors)
2011. ISBN: 978-1-61209-710-7 (Hardcover)
2011. ISBN: 978-1-62417-366-0 (eBook)

Drug Abuse in Hong Kong: Development and Evaluation of a Prevention Program
Daniel TL Shek, Rachel CF Sun and Joav Merrick (Editors)
2011. ISBN: 978-1-61324-491-3 (Hardcover)
2011. ISBN: 978-1-62257-232-8 (eBook)

Chance Action and Therapy: The Playful Way of Changing
Uri Wernik
2010. ISBN: 978-1-60876-393-1 (Hardcover)
2011. ISBN: 978-1-61122-987-5 (Softcover)
2011. ISBN: 978-1-61209-874-6 (eBook)

Bone and Brain Metastases: Advances in Research and Treatment
Arjun Sahgal, Edward Chow and Joav Merrick (Editors)
2010. ISBN: 978-1-61668-365-8 (Hardcover)
2010. ISBN: 978-1-61728-085-6 (eBook)

Children and Pain
Patricia Schofield and Joav Merrick (Editors)
2009. ISBN: 978-1-60876-020-6 (Hardcover)
2009. ISBN: 978-1-61728-183-9 (eBook)

Challenges in Adolescent Health: An Australian Perspective
David Bennett, Susan Towns, Elizabeth Elliott and Joav Merrick (Editors)
2009. ISBN: 978-1-60741-616-6 (Hardcover)
2009. ISBN: 978-1-61668-240-8 (eBook)

Obesity and Adolescence: A Public Health Concern
Hatim A Omar, Donald E Greydanus, Dilip R Patel and Joav Merrick (Editors)
2009. ISBN: 978-1-60692-821-9 (Hardcover)
2009. ISBN: 978-1-61470-465-2 (eBook)

Poverty and Children: A Public Health Concern
Alexis Lieberman and Joav Merrick (Editors)
2009. ISBN: 978-1-60741-140-6 (Hardcover)
2009. ISBN: 978-1-61470-601-4 (eBook)

Living on the Edge: The Mythical, Spiritual, and Philosophical Roots of Social Marginality
Joseph Goodbread
2009. ISBN: 978-1-60741-162-8 (Hardcover)
2013. ISBN: 978-1-61122-986-8 (Softcover)
2011. ISBN: 978-1-61470-192-7 (eBook)

Alcohol-Related Cognitive Disorders: Research and Clinical Perspectives
Leo Sher, Isack Kandel and Joav Merrick (Editors)
2009. ISBN: 978-1-60741-730-9 (Hardcover)
2009. ISBN: 978-1-60876-623-9 (eBook)

Complementary Medicine Systems: Comparison and Integration
Karl W Kratky
2008. ISBN: 978-1-60456-475-4 (Hardcover)
2008. ISBN: 978-1-61122-433-7 (eBook)

Pain in Children and Youth
Patricia Schofield and Joav Merrick (Editors)
2008. ISBN: 978-1-60456-951-3 (Hardcover)
2008. ISBN: 978-1-61470-496-6 (eBook)

Adolescent Behavior Research: International Perspectives
Joav Merrick and Hatim A Omar (Editors)
2007. ISBN: 978-1-60021-649-7

HEALTH AND HUMAN DEVELOPMENT

MEXICO

HEALTH AND AGING

SUPA PENGPID, DrPH
KARL PELTZER, PHD
AND
JOAV MERRICK, MD, MMedSci, DMSc
EDITORS

nova
Medicine & Health
New York

Library of Congress Cataloging-in-Publication Data

Names: Pengpid, Supa, editor. | Peltzer, Karl, editor. | Merrick, Joav, 1950- editor.
Title: Mexico: health and aging / Supa Pengpid, Karl Peltzer, Joav Merrick, editors.
Identifiers: LCCN 2020018266 (print) | LCCN 2020018267 (ebook) | ISBN 9781536179507 (paperback) | ISBN 9781536179514 (adobe pdf)
Subjects: LCSH: Older people--Health and hygiene--Mexico. | Older people--Mental health--Mexico. | Older people--Drug use--Mexico. | Aging--Health aspects--Mexico.
Classification: LCC RA564.8 .M49 2020 (print) | LCC RA564.8 (ebook) | DDC 613/.04380972--dc23
LC record available at https://lccn.loc.gov/2020018266
LC ebook record available at https://lccn.loc.gov/2020018267

Published by Nova Science Publishers, Inc. † New York

CONTENTS

INTRODUCTION

In: Mexico: Health and Aging
Editors: Supa Pengpid et al.
ISBN: 978-1-53617-950-7

Chapter 1

AGEING AND HEALTH IN MEXICO

Supa Pengpid[1,2,*], DrPH, Karl Peltzer[2], PhD and Joav Merrick[3-6], MD, MMedSci, DMSc

[1]ASEAN Institute for Health Development, Mahidol University, Salaya, Phutthamonthon, Nakhon Pathom, Thailand
[2]Department of Research Administration and Development, University of Limpopo, Turfloop, South Africa
[3]National Institute of Child Health and Human Development, Jerusalem, Israel
[4]Department of Pediatrics, Mt Scopus Campus, Hadassah Hebrew University Medical Center, Jerusalem, Israel
[5]Kentucky Children's Hospital, University of Kentucky, Lexington, Kentucky, United States
[6]Center for Healthy Development, School of Public Health, Georgia State University, Atlanta, United States

* Correspondence: Professor Supa Pengpid, ASEAN Institute for Health Development, Mahidol University, 25/25 Phutthamonthon Road 4, Salaya, Phutthamonton, Nakhon Pathom 73170, Thailand. E-Mail: supaprom@yahoo.com.

Abstract

In this book we wanted to identify trajectories of health and their associations with lifestyle factors in a national representative cohort study of older Mexicans. We used secondary data from the Study of Global Ageing and Adult Health (SAGE) second wave 2014-15 in Mexico. The average healthy life expectancy of older Mexicans has actually declined over the past decade. Limited access to nutrition resources and unhealthy dietary styles, due to high poverty, have led to increasing chronic diseases like diabetes among older Mexican adults, which in turn create further financial problems as a result of high out-of-pocket expenditure on healthcare. This book deals with angina pectoris, stroke, oral health, eye health, alcohol use, tobacco use, depression, loneliness, arthritis, back pain, obesity, fruit and vegetable consumption, and sleep. We hope that findings from these papers may aid public policy and programmes for older adults in Mexico.

Introduction

"Mexico's population age 65 years and older is projected to grow by 277 percent from 8.2 million in 2015 to over 30 million by 2050. This rate of growth can be compared with the growth rate of 194 percent for upper-middle-income countries and just 71 percent for high-income countries" (1). "Older Mexican adults' average healthy life expectancy has actually declined over the past decade. Limited access to nutrition resources and unhealthy dietary styles, due to high poverty, have led to increasing chronic diseases like diabetes among older Mexican adults, which in turn create further financial problems as a result of high out-of-pocket expenditure on healthcare" (1).

In this study, we aimed to identify trajectories of health and their associations with lifestyle factors in a national representative cohort study of older Mexicans. We used secondary data of Study of Global Ageing and Adult Health (SAGE) second wave 2014-15 in Mexico (2). The multi-country SAGE is run by the World Health Organization's Multi-Country Studies unit in the Health Systems and Innovation Cluster. SAGE is part of the unit's Longitudinal Study Programme which is compiling longitudinal data on the health and well-being of adult populations, and the ageing process, through primary data collection and secondary data analysis (2). This book deals with angina pectoris, stroke, oral health, eye health, alcohol use, tobacco use, depression, loneliness, arthritis, back pain, obesity, fruit and vegetable consumption, and sleep. We hope that findings from these papers may aid public policy and programmes for older adults in Mexico.

REFERENCES

[1] FP Analytics. The aging readiness and competitiveness report Mexico, 2019. UTL: https://arc.aarpinternational.org/File%20Library/Full%20Reports/ARC-Report---Mexico.pdf.

[2] World Health Organisation. Mexico: Study on global ageing and adult health, 2014, Wave 2. URL: http://apps.who.int/healthinfo/systems/surveydata/index.php/catalog/212/datafile/F2/?offset=1000&limit=100.

SECTION ONE: MEXICO AND HEALTH

In: Mexico: Health and Aging
Editors: Supa Pengpid et al.
ISBN: 978-1-53617-950-7

Chapter 2

PREVALENCE AND CORRELATES OF OBESITY AMONG OLDER ADULTS IN MEXICO: A NATIONAL CROSS-SECTIONAL SURVEY

Supa Pengpid[1,2]***, DrPH and Karl Peltzer***[2,*]***, PhD***
[1]ASEAN Institute for Health Development, Mahidol University, Salaya, Phutthamonthon, Nakhon Pathom, Thailand
[2]Department of Research Administration and Development, University of Limpopo, Turfloop, South Africa

ABSTRACT

In this chapter we aimed to determine the prevalence and correlates of obesity in older Mexicans. The study is based on a national population-based cross-sectional survey of older adults (50 years and older) (SAGE wave 2-2014-15) in Mexico. Weight and height were measured and body mass index (BMI) calculated. The sample included 3,903 older adults (50 years and older), with a median age of 61 years. Results indicate that

* Correspondence: Professor Karl Peltzer, Department of Research Administration and Development, University of Limpopo, Turfloop Campus, Private Bag X1106, Sovenga 0727, South Africa. Email: kfpeltzer@gmail.com.

0.8% of the participants were underweight, 21.9% had normal weight, 41.7% were overweight and 35.5% obese. In adjusted logistic regression analyses, younger age, being female, low and highest wealth status, physical inactivity, and hypertension were associated with obesity. A high prevalence of overweight and obesity was found among older adults in Mexico. Several risk factors were identified, which can be targeted in public health interventions.

INTRODUCTION

Globally, in 2016, "39% of adults aged 18 years and over (39% of men and 40% of women) were overweight and 13% (11% of men and 15% of women)" (1). In 2013 in 10 European countries, the prevalence of obesity among older adults (50 years and older) was 19.2% (2). In the 2006 Mexico "National Health and Nutrition Survey" (60 years or older) the prevalence of overweight and obesity was 42.1% and 29.7%, respectively (3). In the 2009/10 Mexico "Study on Global AGEing and Adult Health (SAGE Wave 1)" among individuals aged 50 years and older, the prevalence of overweight and obesity was 49.4% and 28.7%, respectively (4), and in the 2012 Mexico "National Health and Nutrition Survey" among persons 60 years and older, the prevalence of obesity was 37.3% among women and 21.9% among men (5). There is a lack of more recent data on the national prevalence of obesity and its correlates among older adults in Mexico.

Risk factors for obesity may include sociodemographic factors, lifestyle variables and chronic conditions (6). Sociodemographic factors associated with obesity may include younger age (3, 4), being female (3, 6), married (3), higher educational level (3, 7), higher income (7), and residing in urban areas (3, 4). Life style factors include poor dietary behaviour (6, 8, 9) and physical inactivity (4, 6, 10), and chronic health conditions such as hypertension (6, 11), angina and diabetes (10-12), arthritis (6, 12), stroke (12), and functional disability (12, 13). This aim of this investigation was to report on the prevalence and correlates of obesity in older Mexicans who took part in SAGE wave 2 in 2014.

OUR STUDY

The study is based on a national population-based cross-sectional survey of older adults (50 years and older) (SAGE wave 2-2014-15) in Mexico. The dataset is publically available and study procedures and sampling strategy have been described in detail (14). Briefly, a "stratified multistage cluster sampling design" was used to generate a sample that is nationally representative. Strata were defined by locality (metropolitan, urban, rural). The "Basic Geo-Statistical Areas (AGEB) defined by the National Institute of Statistics (INEGI) constituted the primary sampling units (PSUs) and were selected with probability proportional to size"(14). The individual study response rate was 81% (14).

Household weights (variable hhweight) for analysis at household level and individual weights (variable pweight) for analysis at person level were calculated. These were based on the selection probability at each stage of selection. Household weights were post-stratified by locality according to the 2009 population census projections. Individual weights were post-stratified by sex and age-groups according to the 2009 population census projections. Weights are divided by 1000 and are not normalized (14).

All procedures performed in studies involving human participants were in accordance with the ethical standards of the Research and Ethics Committees of Mexico's National Institute of Public Health and with the 1964 Helsinki declaration and its later amendments or comparable ethical standards. Informed consent was obtained from all individual participants included in the study (14).

Measures

Anthropometry

Weight and height were measured using standard procedures. Body mass index (BMI) was calculated and obesity defined as $\geq$30 kg/m^2 (BMI) (15).

Sociodemographic variables included educational level, marital status, age, sex, residence status and wealth quartiles were calculated based on a 19-item household asset list (using principal component analysis) (16).

Self-rated health status was classified, based on the question "In general, how would you rate your health today?" into poor (bad or very bad), moderate (moderate) and good (good or very good).

Functional ability was measured by the "12-item WHO Disability Assessment Schedule, version 2 (WHODAS-II)" (17), with scores of 25-100 indicating moderate, severe or extreme functional disability (18) (Cronbach alpha 0.90).

Fruit and vegetable (FV) consumption was assessed with two questions: "How many servings of fruits do you eat on a typical day?" and "How many servings of vegetables do you eat on a typical day?" Inadequate FV intake was defined as "less than 5 servings of fruits and/or vegetables a day" (19) (Cronbach alpha 0.65).

Physical activity levels (low, moderate or high) were assessed with the "Global Physical Activity Questionnaire (GPAQ)," it gathers data on three domains of physical activity ("activity at work, travel to and from places, recreational activities") and sedentary behaviour (20).

Sedentary behaviour was measured with one question by the GPAQ on the "time usually spent sitting or reclining on a typical day." Eight or more hours a day was classified as sedentary behaviour (21).

Current and past daily tobacco use was assessed with the questions, "Do you currently use (smoke, sniff or chew) any tobacco products such as cigarettes, cigars, pipes, chewing tobacco or snuff?" and "In the past, did you ever smoke tobacco or use smokeless tobacco daily?"(22).

Current alcohol use was assessed with past month consumption of drinks that "contain alcohol (such as beer, wine, spirits, etc.)."

Hypertension was measured based on the average of two blood pressure measurements and defined as "systolic blood pressure greater than or equal to 140 mmHg and/or diastolic blood pressure greater than or equal to 90 mmHg19 and/or self-reported treatment of hypertension with antihypertensive medication currently (the last two weeks before interview)" (23).

Depression was assessed with asking about depression symptoms in the past 12 months using the "World Mental Health Survey version of the Composite International Diagnostic Interview" (24). Additionally, persons who reported to have taken "any medications or other treatment such as attending therapy or counselling sessions for depression during the last 12 months?" were included in the symptom-based depression.

Diabetes and stroke were assessed by self-reported diagnosis.

Angina was assessed with the "World Health Organization's Rose angina questionnaire" (25).

Arthritis was assessed with a symptom-based algorithm (26).

Data analysis

Considering the clustered study design, data analyses were conducted with "STATA software version 15.0 (Stata Corporation, College Station, TX, USA)." Unadjusted and adjusted logistic regression identified predictors of obesity. P values of below 0.05 were accepted as significant and missing values were excluded from the analysis.

FINDINGS

The sample included 3,903 older adults (50 years and older), with a median age of 61 years (15 years interquartile range), 55.7% were female and 44.3% male. About one-third of the participants (31.1%) had secondary or more education, 66.5% were married or cohabiting, 78.8% were residing in urban areas, 42.1% rated their health status as good, 15.6% had a functional disability, 85.0% ate inadequate fruit and vegetables, 46.7% were physically inactive, and 5.9% engaged in sedentary behaviour. Almost one in ten of the older adults (7.5%) were past and 7.5% were current daily tobacco users, 14.4% consumed alcohol currently, 56.9% had hypertension, 11.6% depression, 23.1% diabetes, 6.4% angina, 3.1% stroke and 14.8% arthritis.

Regarding body weight status, 0.8% were underweight, 21.9% had normal weight, 41.7% were overweight and 35.5% obese (see Table 1).

Table 1. Body weight based on Body Mass Index and chronic disease conditions and lifestyle by gender

Variable	Total sample	Male	Female
	N (%)	%	%
Total sample	3903	44.3	55.7
Body Mass Index (BMI)			
Underweight (BMI <18.5)	35 (0.8)	0.8	0.9
Normal (BMI 18.5-<25.0)	834 (21.9)	27.0	17.9
Pre-obese (BMI 25.0 - 29.9 kg/m²)	1420 (41.7)	44.9	39.1
Class I obese (BMI 30.0 - 34.9 kg/m²)	812 (25.0)	21.6	27.8
Class II obese (BMI 35.0 - 39.9 kg/m²)	216 (7.4)	4.2	9.9
Class III obese (BMI > 40 kg/m²)	104 (3.1)	1.5	4.4
Socio-demographics			
Age in years			
50-59	985 (45.1)	46.0	44.4
60-69	1424 (29.1)	28.6	29.4
70+	1494 (25.8)	25.4	26.1
Education			
<primary	1950 (41.9)	39.6	43.8
primary	986 (27.0)	24.7	28.9
secondary or more	967 (31.1)	35.7	27.4
Marital status			
Single/separated/divorced/widowed	1525 (33.5)	20.1	44.3
Married/cohabitating	2378 (66.5)	79.9	55.7
Wealth quartile			
Lowest	954 (21.6)	22.2	21.2
Low	993 (25.8)	23.4	27.7
High	1004 (26.2)	27.1	25.5
Highest	950 (26.4)	27.3	25.6
Residence			
Rural	1055 (21.2)	23.7	19.1
Urban	2848 (78.8)	76.3	80.9
Health and risk factors			
Subjective health status			
Poor	348 (7.9)	6.8	8.8
Moderate	1898 (50.0)	46.9	52.5
Good	1657 (42.1)	46.3	38.7
Functional disability	643 (15.6)	11.7	18.6
Inadequate fruit and vegetable intake	3293 (85.0)	87.5	82.9

Variable	**Total sample**	**Male**	**Female**
	N (%)	%	%
Physical activity			
Low	1966 (46.7)	42.4	50.0
Moderate	1007 (25.4)	24.5	26.1
High	930 (27.9)	33.1	23.9
Sedentary behaviour	278 (5.9)	8.4	5.3
Past daily tobacco use	294 (6.4)	10.5	3.2
Current daily tobacco user	266 (7.5)	11.7	4.1
Current alcohol use	492 (14.4)	25.2	5.8
Hypertension	2246 (56.9)	54.9	58.6
Depression	442 (11.6)	6.6	15.5
Diabetes	944 (23.1)	21.9	24.0
Angina	253 (6.4)	5.4	7.2
Stroke	127 (3.1)	3.6	2.6
Arthritis	570 (14.8)	11.6	17.3

Associations with obesity

In adjusted logistic regression analyses, younger age, being female, low and highest wealth status, physical inactivity, and hypertension were associated with obesity (see Table 2).

Table 2. The estimated crude odds ratio (OR) of the risk of obesity (based on BMI) and age adjusted odds ratio with socio-demographic, chronic conditions and lifestyle factors

	Crude OR (95%CI)	**Adjusted OR (95% CI)**
Socio-demographics		
Age in years		
50-59	1 (Reference)	1 (Reference)
60-69	0.66 (0.50, 0.87)**	0.55 (0.41, 0.74)***
70+	0.42 (0.32, 0.56)***	0.32 (0.24, 0.43)***
Gender		
Female	1 (Reference)	1 (Reference)
Male	0.52 (0.41, 0.69)***	0.59 (0.46, 0.76)***
Education		
<primary	1 (Reference)	1 (Reference)
primary	1.36 (1.04, 1.78)*	1.03 (0.78, 1.37)
secondary or more	1.32 (1.00, 1.75)	0.99 (0.73, 1.36)

Table 2. (Continued)

	Crude OR (95%CI)	Adjusted OR (95% CI)
Socio-demographics		
Marital status		
Single/separated/divorced/widowed	1 (Reference)	---
Married/cohabitating	1.21 (0.95, 1.55)	
Wealth quartile		
Lowest	1 (Reference)	1 (Reference)
Low	1.84 (1.26, 2.70)**	1,60 (1.09, 2.37)*
High	1.51 (1.00, 2.29)	1.38 (0.93, 2.03)
Highest	1.98 (1.37, 2.85)***	1.79 (1,19, 2,69)**
Residence		
Rural	1 (Reference)	1 (Reference)
Urban	1.43 (1.04, 1.97)*	1.25 (0.88, 1.77)
Health and risk factors		
Subjective health status		
Poor	1 (Reference)	---
Moderate	1.44 (0.92, 2.27)	
Good	1.17 (0.75, 1.84)	
Functional disability	1.26 (0.93, 1.72)	---
Inadequate fruit and vegetable intake	0.74 (0.54, 1.02)	---
Physical activity		
Low	1 (Reference)	1 (Reference)
Moderate	0.88 (0.67, 1.16)	0.88 (0.66, 1.18)
High	0.71 (0.54, 0.94)*	0.75 (0.58, 0.99)*
Sedentary behaviour	1.47 (0.89, 2.42)	---
Past daily tobacco use	0.55 (0.36, 0.85)**	0.71 (0,43, 1.17)
Current daily tobacco user	0.55 (0.32, 0.95)*	0.60 (0.36, 1.00)
Current alcohol use	0.64 (0.42, 0.98)*	0.73 (0.49, 1.09)
Hypertension	1.58 (1.17, 2.13)**	1.95 (1.43, 2.66)***
Depression	1.41 (0.97, 2.07)	---
Diabetes	1.00 (0.73, 1.30)	---
Angina	1.46 (0.96, 2.21)	---
Stroke	1.53 (0.65, 3.59)	---
Arthritis	1.52 (1.10, 2.09)*	1.36 (0.97, 1.88)

DISCUSSION

The study found in a nationally representative sample of older adults (50 years and above) in Mexico in 2014, a high prevalence of overweight (41.7%) and obesity (35.5%), which is much higher than in a study among persons 50 years and older in ten European countries (2), but seems similar to older national surveys in Mexico (3-5).

In agreement with previous studies (3, 4, 6, 7), this investigation found that younger age, female sex and higher wealth levels were associated with obesity. Previous studies in Mexico (3, 4) found that urban residence and higher educational levels were associated with obesity, while in this study similar results were found in unadjusted analysis.

Consistent with previous studies (4, 6, 10), this study showed that physical inactivity was associated with obesity. While poor dietary behaviour (inadequate fruit and vegetable intake) was not significantly associated with obesity, this was found in some former research (8, 9). Regarding chronic conditions, this study discovered that hypertension and in unadjusted analysis arthritis were positively associated with obesity. Similar results were found previously (6, 11, 12). Further, in unadjusted analysis past and current daily tobacco use were protective against obesity, which may be attributed to the appetite-suppressant effect of nicotine or caffeine (27).

Study limitations include the cross-sectional design and the assessment of some variables by self-report.

Conclusion

A high prevalence of overweight and obesity was found among older adults in Mexico, and several associated factors were identified, such as younger age, being female, low and highest wealth status, physical inactivity and hypertension, that could assist in programmes preventing and controlling overweight and obesity.

Acknowledgment

This paper uses data from WHO's Study on Global Ageing and Adult Health (SAGE). SAGE is supported by the US National Institute on Aging through Interagency Agreements OGHA 04034785; YA1323-08-CN-0020; Y1-AG-1005-0) and through research grants R01-AG034479 and R21-AG034263.

References

[1] World Health Organization.Obesity and overweight, 2018. URL: https://www.who.int/news-room/fact-sheets/detail/obesity-and-overweight.

[2] Peralta M, Ramos M, Lipert A, Martins J, Marques A. Prevalence and trends of overweight and obesity in older adults from 10 European countries from 2005 to 2013. Scand J Public Health 2018;46(5):522-9. doi: 10.1177/1403494818764810.

[3] Rosas-Carrasco O, Juarez-Cedillo T, Ruiz-Arregui L, Garcia Pena C, Vargas-Alarcon G, Sánchez-García S. Overweight and obesity as markers for the evaluation of disease risk in older adults. J Nutr Health Aging 2012;16(1):14-20.

[4] Rivas-Marino G, Negin J, Salinas-Rodríguez A, Manrique-Espinoza B, Sterner KN, Snodgrass J, et al. Prevalence of overweight and obesity in older Mexican adults and its association with physical activity and related factors: An analysis of the study on global ageing and adult health. Am J Hum Biol 2015;27(3):326-33. doi: 10.1002/ajhb.22642.

[5] López-Ortega M, Arroyo P. Anthropometric characteristics and body composition in Mexican older adults: age and sex differences. Br J Nutr 2016;115(3):490-9. doi: 10.1017/S0007114515004626.

[6] Peltzer K, Phaswana-Mafuya N, Ramlagan S. Prevalence of obesity and associated factors in South Africans 50 years and older: a brief report. Afr J Phys Health Educ Recreat Dance 2011;17(4):772-778.

[7] Puoane T, Steyn K, Bradshaw D, Laubscher R, Fourie J, Lambert V, et al. Obesity in South Africa: the South African demographic and health survey. Obes Res 2002;10(10):1038-48.

[8] Pengpid S, Peltzer K. The prevalence of underweight, overweight/obesity and their related lifestyle factors in Indonesia, 2014-2015. AIMS Public Health 2017;4(6):633-49. doi: 10.3934/publichealth.2017.6.633.

[9] Cohen SA, Greaney ML, Sabik NJ. Assessment of dietary patterns, physical activity and obesity from a national survey: Rural-urban health disparities in older adults. PLoS One 2018;13(12):e0208268. doi: 10.1371/journal.pone.0208268.

[10] Biritwum RB, Gyapong J, Mensah G. The epidemiology of obesity in Ghana. Ghana Med J 2005;39(3):82-5.

[11] Ahn S, Zhao H, Tai-Seale M, Huber C Jr, Smith ML, Ory MG, et al. The longitudinal effects of behavioral, health, and socio-demographic factors on body

mass index among older Chinese adults. Int J Public Health 2012;57(2):269-77. doi: 10.1007/s00038-011-0249-5.
[12] Erem C, Arslan C, Hacihasanoglu A, Deger O, Topbas M, Ukinc K, et al. Prevalence of obesity and associated risk factors in Turkish population (trabzon city, Turkey). Obes Res 2004;12(7):1117-27.
[13] Samper-Ternent R, Al Snih S. Obesity in older adults: Epidemiology and implications for disability and disease. Rev Clin Gerontol 2012;22(1):10-34.
[14] Kumar A, Karmarkar AM, Tan A, Graham JE, Arcari CM, Ottenbacher KJ, et al. The effect of obesity on incidence of disability and mortality in Mexicans aged 50 years and older. Salud Publica Mex 2015;57(Suppl 1):S31-8.
[15] World Health Organisation. Mexico: Study on global ageing and adult health, 2014, Wave 2. URL: http://apps.who.int/healthinfo/systems/surveydata/index.php/catalog/212/datafile/F2/?offset=1000&limit=100.
[16] World Health Organization. The international classification of adult underweight, overweight and obesity according to BMI, 2018. URL: http://apps.who.int/bmi/index.jsp?introPage=intro_3.html.
[17] Filmer D, Pritchett LH. Estimating wealth effects without expenditure data—or tears: an application to educational enrollments in states of India. Demography 2001;38(1):115–32.
[18] Ustün T, Kostanjsek N, Chatterji S, Rehm J, eds. Measuring health and disability: Manual for WHO disability assessment schedule (WHODAS 2.0) Geneva, Switzerland: WHO, 2010.
[19] World Health Organisation. World report on disability. Malta: WHO, 2011.
[20] World Health Organization. Diet, nutrition, and the prevalence of chronic diseases. Geneva, Switzerland: WHO, 2003.
[21] Bull FC, Maslin TS, Armstrong T. Global physical activity questionnaire (GPAQ): nine country reliability and validity study. J Phys Act Health 2009;6(6):790–804.
[22] Chau JY, Grunseit AC, Chey T, Stamatakis E, Brown WJ, Matthews CE, et al. Daily sitting time and all-cause mortality: a meta-analysis. PLoS One 2013;8(11):e80000.
[23] World Health Organization. Guidelines for controlling and monitoring the tobacco epidemic. Geneva, Switzerland: WHO, 1998.
[24] Chobanian AV, Bakris GL, Black HR, Cushman WC, Green LA, Izzo Jr JL, et al. The seventh report of the joint national committee on prevention, detection, evaluation, and treatment of high blood pressure: the JNC 7 report. JAMA 2003;289(19):2560–71.
[25] Kessler RC, Ustün TB. The World Mental Health (WMH) Survey initiative version of the World Health Organization (WHO) Composite International Diagnostic Interview (CIDI). Int J Methods Psychiatr Res 2004;13(2):93–121.
[26] Rose GA. The diagnosis of ischaemic heart pain and intermittent claudication in field surveys. Bull World Health Organ 1962;27:645–58.
[27] Arokiasamy P, Uttamacharya, Kowal P, Capistrant BD, Gildner TE, Thiele E, et al. Chronic noncommunicable diseases in 6 low- and middle-income countries: findings

from wave 1 of the world health organization's Study on Global Ageing and Adult Health (SAGE). Am J Epidemiol 2017;185(6):414e428. https://doi.org/10.1093/aje/kww125.

[28] Jessen A, Buemann B, Toubro S, Skovgaard IM, Astrup A. The appetite-suppressant effect of nicotine is enhanced by caffeine. Diabetes Obes Metab 2005;7(4):327-33.

In: Mexico: Health and Aging
Editors: Supa Pengpid et al.
ISBN: 978-1-53617-950-7

Chapter 3

PREVALENCE AND CORRELATES OF FRUIT AND VEGETABLE INTAKE AMONG OLDER ADULTS IN MEXICO

Karl Peltzer*[1], *PhD and Supa Pengpid*[1,2,*], *DrPH

[1]Department of Research Administration and Development, University of Limpopo, Turfloop, South Africa

[2]ASEAN Institute for Health Development, Mahidol University, Salaya, Phutthamonthon, Nakhon Pathom, Thailand

ABSTRACT

In this chapter we determine the prevalence and correlates of inadequate fruit and vegetable (FV) consumption in older Mexicans. The study is based on a national population-based cross-sectional survey of older adults (50 years and older) (SAGE wave 2-2014-15) in Mexico. Fruit and vegetable intake were measured with standard procedures. The sample included 3,903 older adults (50 years and older), with a median age of 61

* Correspondence: Professor Supa Pengpid, ASEAN Institute for Health Development, Mahidol University, 25/25 Phutthamonthon Road 4, Salaya, Phutthamonton, Nakhon Pathom 73170, Thailand. Email: supaprom@yahoo.com.

years. Results indicate that the prevalence of inadequate FV intake was 85.0%, 87.5% in men and 82.9% in women, and the mean FV intake per day was 2.9 (SD = 1.8) servings. In adjusted logistic regression analysis, male sex, moderate food insecurity, and high physical activity were positively and highest wealth status and high social engagement were negatively associated with inadequate FV intake. A high prevalence of inadequate FV intake was discovered among older adults in Mexico. Several risk factors were identified, which can be targeted in public health interventions.

INTRODUCTION

Low fruit and vegetable (FV) consumption significantly contributes to morbidity and mortality globally (1). Globally, 78.5% of adult women and 77.6% of adult men consume inadequate FV (<five servings, <400 g) (2). In the 2006 "Mexican National Health and Nutrition Survey" average FV intake was 122.6 g in adults and less than "30% of the Mexican population had adequate intakes of FV" (3). The "National Academy of Medicine of México recommends daily consumption of three portions of vegetables and two portions of fruits." (4) National Academy of Medicine.

Older age may be accompanied with changes, such as in appetite and oral health that could reduce FV intake (5, 6). In a recent review, it was estimated from major studies that only "21 to 37% of men and 29 to 45% of women aged 65 and older achieve the recommended servings per day" (5). In a 2014 study among 948 adults (≥60 years) in Mexico, "routine consumption of fruits and vegetables was reported by 53.8% of older adults" (7). In the 2009-2010 "Study on Global AGEing and Health (SAGE)" among older adults (50 years and older) in Mexico, the prevalence of inadequate FV was 81.4% (8). There seems to be a lack of recent national information on inadequate FV intake among older adults in Mexico.

As reviewed previously (9), factors associated with inadequate FV intake include, "male, sex, older age, lower education, lower income, residence status, lack of social cohesion, being single, widowed or divorced, diabetes, hypertension, overweight or obese, depressive symptoms, poor subjective health status, smoking, physical activity status, alcohol use status and knowledge and psychosocial determinants." This study aimed to determine the prevalence and correlates of inadequate FV consumption in older Mexicans who took part in SAGE wave 2 in 2014.

OUR STUDY

The study is based on a national population-based cross-sectional survey of older adults (50 years and older) (SAGE wave 2-2014-15) in Mexico. The dataset is publically available and study procedures and sampling strategy have been described in detail (10). Briefly, a "stratified multistage cluster sampling design" was used to generate a sample that is nationally representative. Strata were defined by locality (metropolitan, urban, rural). The "Basic Geo-Statistical Areas (AGEB) defined by the National Institute of Statistics (INEGI) constituted the primary sampling units (PSUs) and were selected with probability proportional to size"(10). The individual study response rate was 81% (10).

All procedures performed in studies involving human participants were in accordance with the ethical standards of the Research and Ethics Committees of Mexico's National Institute of Public Health and with the 1964 Helsinki declaration and its later amendments or comparable ethical standards. Informed consent was obtained from all individual participants included in the study (10).

Measures

FV consumption was assessed with two questions: "How many servings of fruits do you eat on a typical day?" and "How many servings of vegetables do you eat on a typical day?" Inadequate FV intake was defined as "less than 5 servings of fruits and/or vegetables a day" (11) (Cronbach alpha 0.65).

Sociodemographic variables included educational level, marital status, age, sex, residence status and wealth quartiles were calculated based on a 19-item household asset list (using principal component analysis) (12).

Self-rated health status was classified, based on the question "In general, how would you rate your health today?" into poor (bad or very bad), moderate (moderate) and good (good or very good).

Food insecurity was assessed with two questions: "In the last 12 months, how often did you ever eat less than you felt you should because there wasn't enough food?" and "In the last 12 months, were you ever hungry, but didn't eat because you couldn't afford enough food?" (Cronbach alpha 0.88). Responses were grouped into no or low, moderate and high food insecurity.

Hypertension was measured based on the average of two blood pressure measurements and defined as "systolic blood pressure greater than or equal to 140 mmHg and/or diastolic blood pressure greater than or equal to 90 mmHg19 and/or self-reported treatment of hypertension with antihypertensive medication currently (the last two weeks before interview)" (13).

Diabetes was assessed by self-reported diagnosis.

Anthropometry. Weight and height were measured using standard procedures. Body mass index (BMI) was calculated and obesity defined as ≥ 30 kg/m^2 (BMI) (14).

Depression was assessed with asking about depression symptoms in the past 12 months using the "World Mental Health Survey version of the Composite International Diagnostic Interview" (15). Additionally, persons who reported to have taken "any medications or other treatment such as attending therapy or counselling sessions for depression during the last 12 months?" were included in the symptom-based depression.

Oral health problems were defined as an affirmative response to the question, "During the last 12 months, have you had any problems with your mouth and/or teeth, including problems with swallowing?"

Edentulism was defined as an affirmative response to the question, "Have you lost all of your natural teeth?"

Current daily tobacco use was assessed with the question, "Do you currently use (smoke, sniff or chew) any tobacco products such as cigarettes, cigars, pipes, chewing tobacco or snuff?" (16)

Current alcohol use was assessed with past month consumption of drinks that "contain alcohol (such as beer, wine, spirits, etc.)"

Physical activity levels (low, moderate or high) were assessed with the "Global Physical Activity Questionnaire (GPAQ)," it gathers data on three domains of physical activity ("activity at work, travel to and from places, recreational activities") (17).

Social engagement was measured with nine items on the participation in social activities, e.g., "How often in the last 12 months have you attended any public meeting in which there was discussion of local or school affairs?" Responses ranged from 1 = never to 5 = daily (18). Scores from the nine questions were summed and classified into three groups of low, moderate and high social engagement (Cronbach alpha 0.65).

Quality of life was measured with the the 8-item "WHO Quality of Life (WHOQol)," using a summative model generating an index (19). (Cronbach alpha 0.79).

Data analysis

Considering the clustered study design, data analyses were conducted with "STATA software version 15.0 (Stata Corporation, College Station, TX, USA)." Unadjusted and adjusted logistic regression identified predictors of inadequate FV intake. P values of below 0.05 were accepted as significant and missing values were excluded from the analysis.

FINDINGS

The sample included 3,903 older adults (50 years and older), with a median age of 61 years (15 years interquartile range), 55.7% were female and

Table 1. Sample and inadequate fruit and vegetable intake characteristics

Variable	Sample	Inadequate fruit and vegetable intake		
		All	Male	Female
	N (%)	%	%	%
All	3903	85.0	87.5	82.9
Age in years				
50-59	985 (45.1)	84.4	86.8	82.4
60-69	1424 (29.1)	86.7	88.7	85.1
70+	1494 (25.8)	84.0	87.5	81.3
Education				
<Primary	1950 (41.9)	87.9	90.3	86.2
Primary	986 (27.0)	84.1	86.0	82.7
Secondary or more	967 (31.1)	81.7	85.5	77.8
Marital status				
Single/separated/divorced/widowed	1525 (33.5)	83.6	88.8	81.7
Married/cohabitating	2378 (66.5)	85.7	87.2	83.9
Wealth quartile				
Lowest	954 (21.6)	89.8	93.2	87.0
Low	993 (25.8)	87.1	88.3	86.2
High	1004 (26.2)	85.3	87.4	83.4
Highest	950 (26.4)	78.6	82.3	75.4
Residence				
Rural	1055 (21.2)	88.1	89.3	87.0
Urban	2848 (78.8)	84.1	87.0	82.0
Health and risk factors				
Subjective health status				
Poor	348 (7.9)	88.8	88.9	88.7
Moderate	1898 (50.0)	84.1	85.9	82.9
Good	1657 (42.1)	85.3	89.0	81.7
Food insecurity				
Low	3127 (79.6)	83.2	86.1	80.6
Moderate	535 (13.1)	93.0	94.1	92.3
High	241 (7.3)	89.8	95.8	86.8
Hypertension	2246 (56.9)	83.6	85.1	82.4
Diabetes	944 (23.1)	85.7	87.2	84.6
Obesity	1132 (35.5)	82.1	79.8	83.3
Depression	442 (11.6)	88.1	97.0	85.1
Oral health problems in past 12 months	667 (17.8)	84.8	80.2	87.9
Edentulism	851 (16.6)	84.2	89.9	81.4
Daily tobacco use	294 (7.5)	86.8	86.9	86.7
Alcohol use (past month)	492 (14.4)	84.3	86.0	78.3

Variable	Sample	Inadequate fruit and vegetable intake		
		All	Male	Female
	N (%)	%	%	%
Physical inactivity				
Low	1966 (46.7)	82.5	84.3	84.3
Moderate	1007 (25.4)	83.3	85.9	85.9
High	930 (27.9)	90.6	92.9	92.9
Social engagement				
Low	1418 (38.6)	88.6	89.4	88.1
Moderate	1279 (32.2)	84.7	89.6	80.8
High	1206 (29.2)	80.4	83.4	77.6
	M (SD)		M (SD)	
Quality of Life (range 0-100)	73.4 (9.1)	73.1 (9.1)		

44.3% male. About one-third of the participants (31.1%) had secondary or more education, 66.5% were married or cohabiting, 78.8% were residing in urban areas, 42.1% rated their health status as good, 7.3% had severe food insecurity, and 46.7% were physically inactive. Almost one in ten of the older adults (7.5%) were current daily tobacco users, 14.4% consumed alcohol currently, 56.9% had hypertension, 11.6% depression, 23.1% diabetes, 17.8% had oral health problems, 16.6% had lost all their teeth, and 35.5% were obese. The prevalence of inadequate FV intake was 85.0%, 87.5% in men and 82.9% in women, and the mean FV intake per day was 2.9 (SD = 1.8) servings (see Table 1).

Associations with inadequate fruit and vegetable intake

In adjusted logistic regression analysis, male sex, moderate food insecurity, and high physical activity were positively and highest wealth status and high social engagement were negatively associated with inadequate FV intake (see Table 2).

Table 2. Associations with inadequate fruit and vegetable consumption in older Mexicans

Variable	Unadjusted Odds Ratios (95% CI)	Adjusted Odds Ratios (95% CI)
Age in years		
50-59	1 (Reference)	---
60-69	1.20 (0.89, 1.61)	
70+	0.97 (0.62, 1.51)	
Gender		
Female	1 (Reference)	1 (Reference)
Male	1.45 (1.06, 1.98)*	1.52 (1.12, 2.06)**
Education		
<Primary	1 (Reference)	1 (Reference)
Primary	0.72 (0.53, 0.98)	0.83 (0.59, 1.14)
Secondary or more	0.61 (0.42, 0.89)*	0.87 (0.58, 1.29)
Marital status		
Single/separated/divorced/widowed	1 (Reference)	---
Married/cohabitating	1.17 (0.88, 1.57)	
Wealth quartile		
Lowest	1 (Reference)	1 (Reference)
Low	0.76 (0.45, 1.29)	0.88 (0.52, 1.49)
High	0.65 (0.40, 1.06)	0.81 (0.51, 1.29)
Highest	0.41 (0.25, 0.68)***	0.57 (0.35, 0.92)*
Residence		
Rural	1 (Reference)	---
Urban	0.71 (0.43, 1.19)	
Health and risk factors		
Subjective health status		
Poor	1 (Reference)	---
Moderate	0.67 (0.35, 1.28)	
Good	0.73 (0.38, 1.41)	
Food incesurity		
Low	1 (Reference)	1 (Reference)
Moderate	2.68 (1.59, 4.52)***	2.21 (1.32, 3.69)**
High	1.79 (0.87, 3.66)	1.34 (0.67, 2.69)
Hypertension	0.78 (0.56, 1.07)	---
Diabetes	1.08 (0.79, 1.48)	---
Obesity	0.74 (0.54, 1.02)	---
Depression	1.36 (0.84, 2.20)	---
Oral health problems in past 12 months	0.99 (0.67, 1.46)	---
Edentulism	0.93 (0.66, 1.32)	---
Daily tobacco use	1.18 (0.67, 2.07)	---
Alcohol use (past month)	0.94 (0.60, 1.46)	---

Variable	Unadjusted Odds Ratios (95% CI)	Adjusted Odds Ratios (95% CI)
Physical inactivity		
Low	1 (Reference)	1 (Reference)
Moderate	1.06 (0.75, 1.49)	1.19 (0.82, 1.71)
High	2.03 (1.33, 3.13)***	2.02 (1.31, 3.11)**
Social engagement		
Low	1 (Reference)	1 (Reference)
Moderate	0.71 (0.47, 1.08)	0.72 (0.48, 1.11)
High	0.53 (0.36, 0.77)***	0.52 (0.35, 0.76)***
Quality of Life	0.97 (0.95, 0.99)**	0.98 (0.96, 1.01)

CI = Confidence Interval; ***P < .001; **P < .01; *P < 0.5.

DISCUSSION

In this nationally representative sample of older adults in Mexico, the prevalence of inadequate FV intake was 85.0%, which is higher than in previous studies in Mexico and elsewhere (5, 7, 8). This finding is of concern calling for FV interventions in Mexico. "The main barrier to the consumption of fruits and vegetables in six Latin American countries was the lack of policy support and related public policy, being a good advertising campaign vital to the success of programs that encourage consumption" (20).

Consistent with previous studies (7, 21, 22), this study showed that the prevalence of inadequate FV intake was significantly higher among men than women. Possible reasons for this include that men are less aware than women of FV intake recommendations and its relationship to health and disease (5). As found in previous investigations (2, 5, 7, 9, 21), the results of this investigation showed that higher wealth status, moderate food insecurity and in unadjusted analysis higher educational level was protective against inadequate FV intake. This finding may support the idea that FV costs are a barrier to FV intake of consumers with lower income, and may lent support to programmes in making FV more affordable to the poor (3, 23).

Unlike in some other studies (2, 5, 24), this study did not find any effect of age, marital status, geolocality, substance use and certain chronic conditions on inadequate FV intake. Furthermore, contrary to some previous studies (6), this study did not find that poor oral health and edentulism were associated with inadequate FV intake. Unlike some other studies (21, 25), this study did not find low but high physical activity to be associated with inadequate FV intake. It is possible that persons with lower wealth engage more likely in high physical activity, which may explain this relationship.

Inadequate FV intake among older adults in Mexico may not cluster with health risk behaviours, such as substance use. The study found in agreement with former research (5, 21, 26) that low social engagement or cohesion was associated with inadequate FV intake. The beneficial impact of social engagement on FV intake may be multi-factorial, including social interaction, companionship and socialization (5). Study limitations include the cross-sectional design, the assessment of some variables by self-report, and that certain relevant variables, such as knowledge on FV consumption, were not assessed.

Conclusion

A high prevalence of inadequate FV intake was found among older adults in Mexico, and several associated factors were identified, such as male sex, lower wealth status, moderate food insecurity, low social engagement and high physical activity, that could assist in programmes promoting FV consumption.

Acknowledgments

This paper uses data from WHO's Study on Global Ageing and Adult Health (SAGE). SAGE is supported by the US National Institute on Aging through Interagency Agreements OGHA 04034785; YA1323-08-CN-0020; Y1-AG-1005-0) and through research grants R01-AG034479 and R21-AG034263.

REFERENCES

[1] Yip CSC, Chan W, Fielding R. The associations of fruit and vegetable intakes with burden of diseases: A systematic review of meta-analyses. J Acad Nutr Diet 2019;119(3):464-81. doi: 10.1016/j.jand.2018.11.007.

[2] Hall JN, Moore S, Harper SB, Lynch JW. Global variability in fruit and vegetable consumption. Am J Prev Med 2009;36(5):402-9.

[3] Ramírez-Silva I, Rivera JA, Ponce X, Hernández-Avila M. Fruit and vegetable intake in the Mexican population: results from the Mexican National Health and Nutrition Survey 2006. Salud Publica Mex 2009;51(Suppl 4):S574-85.

[4] National Academy of Medicine. Dietary and physical activity guidelines in the context of overweight and obesity in the Mexican population, 1st ed. Mexico DF: Intersistemas, SA. de CV, 2015.

[5] Nicklett EJ, Kadell AR. Fruit and vegetable intake among older adults: a scoping review. Maturitas 2013;75(4):305-12. doi: 10.1016/j.maturitas.2013.05.005.

[6] Walls AW, Steele JG. The relationship between oral health and nutrition in older people. Mech Ageing Dev 2004;125(12):853–7.

[7] Doubova SV, Sánchez-García S, Infante-Castañeda C, Pérez-Cuevas R. Factors associated with regular physical exercise and consumption of fruits and vegetables among Mexican older adults. BMC Public Health 2016;16:952. doi: 10.1186/s12889-016-3628-2.

[8] Wu F, Guo Y, Chatterji S, Zheng Y, Naidoo N, Jiang Y, et al. Common risk factors for chronic non-communicable diseases among older adults in China, Ghana, Mexico, India, Russia and South Africa: the study on global AGEing and adult health (SAGE) wave 1. BMC Public Health 2015;15:88. doi: 10.1186/s12889-015-1407-0.

[9] Peltzer K, Phaswana-Mafuya N. Fruti and vegetable intake and associated factors in older adults in South Africa. Glob Health Action 2012;5:1-8. doi: 10.3402 /gha.v5i0.18668.

[10] World Health Organisation. Mexico: Study on global ageing and adult health, 2014, Wave 2. URL: http://apps.who.int/healthinfo/systems/surveydata/index.php/catalog/212/datafile/F2/?offset=1000&limit=100.

[11] World Health Organization. Diet, nutrition, and the prevalence of chronic diseases. Geneva, Switzerland: WHO, 2003.

[12] Filmer D, Pritchett LH. Estimating wealth effects without expenditure data—or tears: an application to educational enrollments in states of India. Demography 2001;38(1):115–32.

[13] Chobanian AV, Bakris GL, Black HR, Cushman WC, Green LA, Izzo Jr JL, et al. The seventh report of the joint national committee on prevention, detection, evaluation, and treatment of high blood pressure: the JNC 7 report. JAMA 2003;289(19):2560–71

[14] World Health Organization. The international classification of adult underweight, overweight and obesity according to BMI, 2018. URL: http://apps.who.int/bmi/index.jsp?introPage=intro_3.html.

[15] Kessler RC, Ustün TB. The World Mental Health (WMH) Survey initiative version of the World Health Organization (WHO) Composite International Diagnostic Interview (CIDI). Int J Methods Psychiatr Res 2004;13(2):93–121.

[16] World Health Organization. Guidelines for controlling and monitoring the tobacco epidemic. Geneva, Switzerland: WHO, 1998.

[17] Bull FC, Maslin TS, Armstrong T. Global physical activity questionnaire (GPAQ): nine country reliability and validity study. J Phys Act Health 2009;6(6):790–804.

[18] Kowal P, Chatterji S, Naidoo N, Biritwum R, Fan W, Lopez Ridaura R, et al. Data resource profile: the World Health Organization study on global AGEing and adult health (SAGE). Int J Epidemiol 2012;41(6):1639–49.

[19] Power M. Development of a common instrument for quality of life. In: A. Nosikov and C. Gudex EUROHIS: Developing Common Instruments for Health Surveys. Amsterdam: IOS Press, 2003;57:145-63.

[20] Olavarría S, Zacarías I. Barriers and facilitators to increase consumption of fruits and vegetables in six countries in Latin America. Arch Latinoam Nutr 2011;61(2):154-62.

[21] Li Y, Li D, Ma CY, Liu CY, Hui-Ding, Wen ZM, et al. Consumption and factors influencing consumption of fruit and vegetables among elderly Chinese people. Nutrition 2012;28(5):504-8.

[22] Baker AH, Wardle J. Sex differences in fruit and vegetable intake in older adults. Appetite 2003;40(3):269-75.

[23] Pollard J, Kirk SF, Cade JE. Factors affecting food choice in relation to fruit and vegetable intake: a review. Nutr Res Rev 2002;15(2):373-87.

[24] Li Y, Zhang M, Jiang Y, Wu F. Co-variations and clustering of chronic disease behavioral risk factors in China: China chronic disease and risk factor surveillance, 2007. PLoS One 2012;7(3):e33881.

[25] Sahyoun NR, Zhang XL, Serdula MK. Barriers to the consumption of fruits and vegetables among older adults. J Nutr Elder 2005;24(4):5-21.

[26] Salehi L, Eftekhar H, Mohammad K, Tavafian SS, Jazayery A, Montazeri A. Consumption of fruit and vegetables among elderly people: A cross sectional study from Iran. Nutr J 2010;13;9:2.

In: Mexico: Health and Aging
Editors: Supa Pengpid et al.
ISBN: 978-1-53617-950-7

Chapter 4

PREVALENCE AND CORRELATES OF ORAL HEALTH PROBLEMS AMONG A NATIONALLY REPRESENTATIVE SAMPLE OF OLDER ADULTS IN MEXICO

Supa Pengpid[1,2], DrPH and Karl Peltzer[2,*], PhD
[1]ASEAN Institute for Health Development, Mahidol University, Salaya, Phutthamonthon, Nakhon Pathom, Thailand and [2]Department of Research Administration and Development, University of Limpopo, Turfloop, South Africa

ABSTRACT

In this study we try to determine the prevalence and correlates of oral health problems in older Mexicans. The study is based on a national population-based cross-sectional survey of older adults (50 years and older) (SAGE wave 2-2014-15) in Mexico. Oral health problems were

---

* Correspondence: Professor Karl Peltzer, Department of Research Administration and Development, University of Limpopo, Turfloop Campus, Private Bag X1106, Sovenga 0727, South Africa. Email: kfpeltzer@gmail.com.

assessed by self-report. The sample included 3,903 older adults (50 years and older), with a median age of 61 years. Results indicate that the prevalence of (self-reported) oral health problems was 17.8%, 16.7% in men and 18.8% in women. In adjusted logistic regression analysis, high physical activity, depression and poor self-rated health status were associated with oral health problems. In sex stratified adjusted logistic regression analysis among women, current daily tobacco use was significantly associated with oral health problems. Almost two in five older adults reported oral health problems in Mexico. Several risk factors were identified, which can be targeted in public health interventions.

INTRODUCTION

Oral health is defined by the World Health Organization (WHO) as "a state of being free from mouth and facial pain, oral and throat cancer, oral infection and sores, periodontal (gum) disease, tooth decay, tooth loss, and other diseases and disorders that limit an individual's capacity in biting, chewing, smiling, speaking, and psychosocial well-being" (1). Globally, oral health has deteriorated over the last 25 years "due to demographic changes, including population growth and aging" (2). "Oral diseases are highly prevalent in the globe, posing a very serious public health challenge to policy makers" (2). Globally, poor oral health among older adults is seen by high levels of oral health problems, including "loss of teeth, edentulism, periodontitis, coronal and root caries, oral mucosal lesions, utilization of non-functional dental prostheses, xerostomia, and chewing problems" (3, 4). There is a lack of national population-based data on oral health problems (self-reported) among older adults in Mexico.

In a cross-sectional study of 336 beneficiaries (60 years and older) of social security services in Mexico City, the oral health status was found as not optimal (5). In a community sample of 70 years and older residents (N = 197) in a district of Mexico City, some of the oral health problems included 23.5% edentulism and 8.9% severe periodontitis (4). Further, in a cross-sectional investigation of 139 persons 60 years and older "living in long-term care facilities or living independently and participating in adult day care services in the city of Pachuca, Mexico," the prevalence of oral health problems included edentulism 38.9%, dental caries 95.3% and periodontitis 80% (6).

In national population-based studies in predominantly older adults, the prevalence pf oral health problems was in China 9.3%, India 11.4%, and Russia 35.4% (7). As reviewed previously (7), factors associated with oral health problems include, "age, education, socioeconomic status, sex, residence status, body mass index, smoking, alcohol use, diabetes, hypertension, and coronary heart disease." This study aimed to determine the prevalence and correlates of oral health problems in older Mexicans who took part in SAGE wave 2 in 2014.

OUR STUDY

The study is based on a national population-based cross-sectional survey of older adults (50 years and older) (SAGE wave 2-2014-15) in Mexico. The dataset is publically available and study procedures and sampling strategy have been described in detail (8). Briefly, a "stratified multistage cluster sampling design" was used to generate a sample that is nationally representative. Strata were defined by locality (metropolitan, urban, rural). The "Basic Geo-Statistical Areas (AGEB) defined by the National Institute of Statistics (INEGI) constituted the primary sampling units (PSUs) and were selected with probability proportional to size"(8). The individual study response rate was 81% (8).

All procedures performed in studies involving human participants were in accordance with the ethical standards of the Research and Ethics Committees of Mexico's National Institute of Public Health and with the 1964 Helsinki declaration and its later amendments or comparable ethical standards. Informed consent was obtained from all individual participants included in the study (8).

Measures

Oral health problems were defined as an affirmative response to the question, "During the last 12 months, have you had any problems with your mouth and/or teeth, including problems with swallowing?" (7, 9).

Sociodemographic variables included educational level, age, sex, residence status and wealth quartiles were calculated based on a 19-item household asset list (using principal component analysis) (10).

Anthropometry. Weight and height were measured using standard procedures. Body mass index (BMI) was calculated and overweight and obesity defined as 25.0-29.9 kg/m^2 and ≥ 30 kg/m^2 (BMI), respectively (11).

Current daily tobacco use was assessed with the question, "Do you currently use (smoke, sniff or chew) any tobacco products such as cigarettes, cigars, pipes, chewing tobacco or snuff?" (12).

Current alcohol use was assessed with past month consumption of drinks that "contain alcohol (such as beer, wine, spirits, etc.)".

FV consumption was assessed with two questions: "How many servings of fruits do you eat on a typical day?" and "How many servings of vegetables do you eat on a typical day?" Inadequate FV intake was defined as "less than 5 servings of fruits and/or vegetables a day" (13) (Cronbach alpha 0.65).

Physical activity levels (low, moderate or high) were assessed with the "Global Physical Activity Questionnaire (GPAQ)", it gathers data on three domains of physical activity ("activity at work, travel to and from places, recreational activities") (14).

Hypertension was measured based on the average of two blood pressure measurements and defined as "systolic blood pressure greater than or equal to 140 mmHg and/or diastolic blood pressure greater than or equal to 90 mmHg19 and/or self-reported treatment of hypertension with antihypertensive medication currently (the last two weeks before interview)" (15).

Diabetes and *stroke* were assessed by self-reported diagnosis.

Angina was assessed with the "World Health Organization's Rose angina questionnaire" (16).

Depression was assessed with asking about depression symptoms in the past 12 months using the "World Mental Health Survey version of the Composite International Diagnostic Interview" (17). Additionally, persons who reported to have taken "any medications or other treatment such as attending therapy or counselling sessions for depression during the last 12 months?" were included in the symptom-based depression.

Self-rated health status was classified, based on the question "In general, how would you rate your health today?" into poor (bad or very bad), moderate (moderate) and good (good or very good).

Data analysis

Considering the clustered study design, data analyses were conducted with "STATA software version 15.0 (Stata Corporation, College Station, TX, USA)." Unadjusted and adjusted logistic regression identified predictors of oral health problems. P values of below 0.05 were accepted as significant and missing values were excluded from the analysis

FINDINGS

The sample included 3,903 older adults (50 years and older), with a median age of 61 years (15 years interquartile range), 55.7% were female and 44.3% male. About one-third of the participants (31.1%) had secondary or more education, 78.8% were residing in urban areas, 42.1% rated their health status as good, and 46.7% were physically inactive. Almost one in ten of the older adults (7.5%) were current daily tobacco users, 14.4% consumed alcohol currently, 56.9% had hypertension, 11.6% depression, 23.1% diabetes, 6.4% angina, 3.1% stroke, and 41.7% and 35.5% were overweight and obese, respectively. The prevalence of oral health problems was 17.8%, 16.7% in men and 18.8% in women (see Table 1).

Table 1. Sample and oral health problems characteristics

Variable	Sample	Oral health problems		
		All	Male	Female
	N (%)	%	%	%
All	3903	17.8	16.7	18.8
Age in years				
50-59	985 (45.1)	18.9	17.1	20.4
60-69	1424 (29.1)	17.5	16.9	17.9
70+	1494 (25.8)	16.4	15.6	17.0
Education				
<Primary	1950 (41.9)	17.0	16.8	17.1
Primary	986 (27.0)	20.0	18.5	21.0
Secondary or more	967 (31.1)	17.1	15.3	19.0
Wealth quartile				
Lowest	954 (21.6)	17.5	19.2	16.1
Low	993 (25.8)	18.8	19.0	18.7
High	1004 (26.2)	19.8	17.3	21.9
Highest	950 (26.4)	15.2	11.9	17.9
Residence				
Rural	1055 (21.2)	17.4	18.5	16.4
Urban	2848 (78.8)	17.9	16.1	19.3
Body weight and health risk behaviours				
Body Mass Index				
Normal weight	834 (21.9)	20.2	18.5	22.4
Overweight	1420 (41.7)	16.8	16.3	17.2
Obesity	1132 (35.5)	19.5	16.9	20.9
Daily tobacco use	266 (7.5)	21.8	15.4	36.5
Current alcohol use	492 (14.4)	18.1	16.5	23.5
Inadequate fruit and vegetable intake	3293 (85.0)	17.6	14.9	20.0
Physical inactivity				
Low	1966 (46.7)	15.7	15.5	15.8
Moderate	1007 (25.4)	16.1	13.8	17.8
High	930 (27.9)	23.1	20.4	26.0
Chronic conditions				
Hypertension	2246 (56.9)	16.8	16.0	17.4
Diabetes	944 (23.1)	18.9	19.6	18.4
Angina	253 (6.4)	22.5	21.3	23.3
Stroke	127 (3.1)	19.1	14.0	24.9
Depression	442 (11.6)	29.4	28.2	29.9
Subjective health status				
Poor	348 (7.9)	28.3	28.5	28.2
Moderate	1898 (50.0)	20.1	20.8	19.6
Good	1657 (42.1)	13.2	10.8	15.4

Associations with oral health problems

Table 2. Associations with oral health problems in older Mexicans

Variable	Unadjusted Odds Ratios (95% CI)	Adjusted Odds Ratios (95% CI)
Age in years		
50-59	1 (Reference)	---
60-69	0.91 (0.61, 1.35)	
70+	0.84 (0.61, 1.17)	
Gender		
Female	1 (Reference)	---
Male	0.87 (0.66, 1.14)	
Education		
<Primary	1 (Reference)	---
Primary	1.22 (0.86, 1.73)	
Secondary or more	1.01 (0.72, 1.43)	
Wealth quartile		
Lowest	1 (Reference)	---
Low	1.09 (0.79, 1.52)	
High	1.16 (0.82, 1.64)	
Highest	0.84 (0.59, 1.19)	
Residence		
Rural	1 (Reference)	---
Urban	1.04 (0.77, 1.39)	
Body weight and health risk behaviours		
Body Mass Index		
Normal weight	1 (Reference)	---
Overweight	0.81 (0.52, 1.25)	
Obesity	0.97 (0.66, 1.44)	
Daily tobacco use	1.31 (0.79, 2.19)	---
Current alcohol use	1.02 (0.67, 1.54)	---
Inadequate fruit and vegetable intake	0.99 (0.67, 1.46)	---
Physical inactivity		
Low	1 (Reference)	1 (Reference)
Moderate	1.03 (0.73, 1.45)	1.09 (0.75, 1.57)
High	1.61 (1.16, 2.25)**	1.77 (1.27, 2.46)***
Chronic conditions		
Hypertension	0.82 (0.59, 1.15)	---
Diabetes	1.10 (0.83, 1.45)	---
Angina	1.37 (0.85, 2.20)	---
Stroke	1.09 (0.54, 2.22)	---
Depression	2.14 (1.41, 3.24)***	1.88 (1.22, 2.86)**
Subjective health status		
Poor	1 (Reference)	1 (Reference)
Moderate	0.64 (0.42, 0.96)*	0.72 (0.47, 1.10)
Good	0.38 (0.24, 0.60)***	0.44 (0.28, 0.69)***

CI = Confidence Interval; ***P <. 001; **P < .01; *P < 0.5.

In adjusted logistic regression analysis, high physical activity, depression and poor self-rated health status were associated with oral health problems. In sex stratified adjusted logistic regression analysis among women, current daily tobacco use was significantly associated with oral health problems (OR: 2.70, CI = 1.17, 6.20) (see Table 2).

DISCUSSION

In this nationally representative sample of older adults in Mexico, the prevalence of self-rated oral health problems was 17.8%, which is higher than among predominantly older adults in China (9.3%) and India (11.4%) but lower than in Russia (35.4%) (7). This result confirms findings from different local studies in Mexico, highlighting the importance of oral health problems among older adults in Mexico (4-6).

Consistent with previous studies (18, 19), this study showed that the poor general self-rated health status was associated with a higher prevalence of oral health problems. This investigation found a significant positive association between depression and oral health problems. Results of a "systematic review and meta-analyses show a positive association between depression and oral diseases, specifically dental caries, tooth loss, and edentulism, in adults and elders" (20). Contrary to a study that found beneficial effects of physical activity on oral health (21), this study found a positive association between high physical activity and oral health problems. This result is not clear and requires further studies. Further, this study found among women an association between daily tobacco use and oral health problem. A previous study (22) found that cigarette smoking increased the risk for oral health problems, such as missing teeth, decayed teeth and periodontal disease.

Unlike in some other studies (7), this study did not find any effect of socioeconomic status, sex, residence status, alcohol use, overweight or obesity, hypertension, diabetes, stroke and angina on oral health problems. Study limitations include the cross-sectional design, the assessment of some variables, including oral health status, by self-report, and that certain relevant variables, such as certain dietary behaviours (e.g., sugar and soft drink intake) knowledge on FV consumption, were not assessed.

Conclusion

Almost two in five older adults reported oral health problems in Mexico, and several associated factors were identified, such as poor self-rated health status, depression, tobacco use and high physical activity, that could assist in programmes promoting FV consumption.

Acknowledgment

This paper uses data from WHO's Study on Global Ageing and Adult Health (SAGE). SAGE is supported by the US National Institute on Aging through Interagency Agreements OGHA 04034785; YA1323-08-CN-0020; Y1-AG-1005-0) and through research grants R01-AG034479 and R21-AG034263.

References

[1] Petersen PE, WHO Oral Health Programme. *The world oral health report 2003: Continuous improvement of oral health in the 21st century–the approach of the WHO Global Oral Health Programme*. Geneva: World Health Organization, 2003.

[2] Kassebaum NJ, Smith AGC, Bernabé E, Fleming TD, Reynolds AE, Vos T, et al. Global, regional, and national prevalence, incidence, and disability-adjusted life years for oral conditions for 195 countries, 1990-2015: A systematic analysis for the global burden of diseases, injuries, and risk factors. *J Dent Res* 2017;96(4):380-7. doi: 10.1177/0022034517693566.

[3] Petersen PE, Ueda H. WHO Oral Health Programme and WHO Centre for Health Development (Kobe, Japin :in ageing societies Oral health .Integration of oral health and general health: Report of a meeting convened at the WHO Centre for Health Development in Kobe, Japan, 1-3 June 2005. Geneva: World Health Organization, 2008. URL: https://apps.who.int/iris/handle/10665/43531.

[4] Castrejón-Pérez RC, Borges-Yáñez SA, Gutiérrez-Robledo LM, Avila-Funes JA. Oral health conditions and frailty in Mexican community-dwelling elderly: A cross sectional analysis. *BMC Public Health* 2012;12:773. doi: 10.1186/1471-2458-12-773.

[5] Sánchez-García S, Heredia-Ponce E, Cruz-Hervert P, Juárez-Cedillo T, Cárdenas-Bahena A, García-Peña C. Oral health status in older adults with social security in Mexico City: Latent class analysis. *J Clin Exp Dent* 2014;6(1):e29-35. doi: 10.4317/jced.51224.

[6] Islas-Granillo H, Borges-Yañez SA, Navarrete-Hernández JJ, Veras-Hernández MA, Casanova-Rosado JF, Minaya-Sánchez M, et al. Indicators of oral health in older adults with and without the presence of multimorbidity: A cross-sectional study. *Clin Interv Aging* 2019;14:219-24. doi: 10.2147/CIA.S170470.

[7] Bawankule R, Singh A, Kumar K, Pedgaonkar S. Oral problems and associated risk indicators in adults in the Russian Federation, India, and China. *BMC Oral Health* 2019;19(1):114. doi: 10.1186/s12903-019-0811-8.

[8] World Health Organisation. *Mexico: Study on global ageing and adult health,* 2014, Wave 2. URL: http://apps.who.int/healthinfo/ systems/surveydata/index.php/catalog/212/datafile/F2/?offset=1000&limit=100.

[9] Kowal P, Chatterji S, Naidoo N, Biritwum R, Fan W, Lopez Ridaura R, et al. Data resource profile: the World Health Organization study on global AGEing and adult health (SAGE). *Int J Epidemiol* 2012;41(6):1639–49.

[10] Filmer D, Pritchett LH. Estimating wealth effects without expenditure data—or tears: an application to educational enrollments in states of India. *Demography* 2001;38(1):115–32.

[11] World Health Organization (WHO). *The international classification of adult underweight, overweight and obesity according to BMI, 2018.* URL: http://apps.who.int/bmi/index.jsp?introPage=intro_ 3.html.

[12] World Health Organization. *Guidelines for controlling and monitoring the tobacco epidemic.* Geneva, Switzerland: WHO, 1998.

[13] World Health Organization. *Diet, nutrition, and the prevalence of chronic diseases.* Geneva, Switzerland: WHO, 2003.

[14] Bull FC, Maslin TS, Armstrong T. Global physical activity questionnaire (GPAQ): nine country reliability and validity study. *J Phys Act Health* 2009;6(6):790–804.

[15] Chobanian AV, Bakris GL, Black HR, Cushman WC, Green LA, Izzo Jr JL, et al. The seventh report of the joint national committee on prevention, detection, evaluation, and treatment of high blood pressure: the JNC 7 report. *JAMA* 2003;289(19):2560–71.

[16] Rose GA. The diagnosis of ischaemic heart pain and intermittent claudication in field surveys. *Bull World Health Organ* 1962;27:645–58.

[17] Kessler RC, Ustün TB. The world mental health (WMH) survey initiative version of the World Health Organization (WHO) Composite International Diagnostic Interview (CIDI). *Int J Methods Psychiatr Res* 2004;13(2):93–121.

[18] Brennan DS, Singh KA.General health and oral health self-ratings, and impact of oral problems among older adults. *Eur J Oral Sci* 2011;119(6):469-73. doi: 10.1111/j.1600-0722.2011.00873.x.

[19] Cárdenas-Bahena Á, Velázquez-Olmedo LB, Falcón-Flores JA, García-Zámano IE, Montes-Salmerón RE, Reza-Bravo GG, et al. Self-perception of oral health in older adults from Mexico City. *Rev Med Inst Mex Seguro Soc* 2018;56(Suppl 1):S54-S63.

[20] Cademartori MG, Gastal MT, Nascimento GG, Demarco FF, Corrêa MB. Is depression associated with oral health outcomes in adults and elders? A systematic review and meta-analysis. *Clin Oral Investig* 2018;22(8):2685-2702. doi: 10.1007/s00784-018-2611-y.

[21] Anderson AP, Park YM, Shrestha D, Zhang J, Liu J, Merchant AT. Cross-sectional association of physical activity and periodontal antibodies. *J Periodontol* 2018;89(12):1400-6. doi: 10.1002/JPER.17-0709.

[22] Ide R, Mizoue T, Ueno K, Fujino Y, Yoshimura T. Relationship between cigarette smoking and oral health status. *Sangyo Eiseigaku Zasshi* 2002;44(1):6-11.

In: Mexico: Health and Aging
Editors: Supa Pengpid et al.
ISBN: 978-1-53617-950-7

Chapter 5

PREVALENCE AND CORRELATES OF PAST AND CURRENT TOBACCO USE AMONG A NATIONALLY REPRESENTATIVE SAMPLE OF OLDER ADULTS IN MEXICO

Karl Peltzer[1], PhD and Supa Pengpid[1,2,*], DrPH

[1]Department of Research Administration and Development, University of Limpopo, Turfloop, South Africa and [2]ASEAN Institute for Health Development, Mahidol University, Salaya, Phutthamonthon, Nakhon Pathom, Thailand

ABSTRACT

In this chapter we aimed to determine the prevalence and correlates of past and current tobacco use in older Mexicans. The study is based on a national population-based cross-sectional survey of older adults (50 years and older) (SAGE wave 2-2014-15) in Mexico. Oral health problems

---

Correspondence: Professor Supa Pengpid, ASEAN Institute for Health Development, Mahidol University, 25/25 Phutthamonthon Road 4, Salaya, Phutthamonton, Nakhon Pathom 73170, Thailand. Email: supaprom@yahoo.com.

were assessed by self-report. The sample included 3,903 older adults (50 years and older), with a median age of 61 years. Results indicate that the prevalence of past and current tobacco use was 13.5% and 12.1%, respectively, and among women 7.1% and 6.4% respectively and among men 21.4% and 19.2%, respectively. In adjusted multinomial logistic regression analysis, older age, male sex and urban residence were associated with past tobacco use, and younger age (50-59 years), male sex, urban residence, angina, current alcohol use and low social engagement were positively and functional disability negatively associated with current tobacco use. One in four older adults reported past or current tobacco use in Mexico. Several risk factors were identified, which can be targeted in public health interventions.

INTRODUCTION

Tobacco kills more than eight million people each year; 80% of the world's 1.1 billion smokers live in low- and middle-income countries (1). Smoking is known to cause various illnesses, including cancer, heart disease, stroke, lung diseases, diabetes, and chronic obstructive pulmonary disease (COPD) (2). Older adults seem to continue tobacco use to a high extent and may be more unaware of its harmful effects (3-5). In a study among older adults (50 years and older) in six middle-income countries, the prevalence of current tobacco use ranged from 10.2% in Ghana to 49.4% in India, and in 2009/2010 in Mexico 19.9% (6). In a systematic review on tobacco use among the elderly, the "overall prevalence of tobacco use was 13% in both genders (22% male and 8% female" (3). Based on the "Global Adult Tobacco Survey (GATS) 2008-2010", the prevalence of current tobacco use was 16.1% in Mexico (7). There is a lack of more recent national data on the prevalence and correlates on tobacco use among older adults in Mexico.

As previously reviewed (5), factors associated with "current tobacco use among older adults include age, male sex, lower socioeconomic status, residence status, poor self-rated health, chronic diseases such as chronic obstructive pulmonary disease, mental health difficulties, insufficient fruits and vegetable consumption." In a somewhat similar fashion, factors associated with past tobacco use or tobacco use cessation among older adults include "older age, sex, higher socioeconomic status, urban residence, cardiovascular disorders, asthma angina, and mental health difficulties" (5). This study aimed to determine the prevalence and correlates of tobacco use in older Mexicans who took part in SAGE wave 2 in 2014.

OUR STUDY

The study is based on a national population-based cross-sectional survey of older adults (50 years and older) (SAGE wave 2-2014-15) in Mexico. The dataset is publically available and study procedures and sampling strategy have been described in detail (8). Briefly, a "stratified multistage cluster sampling design" was used to generate a sample that is nationally representative. Strata were defined by locality (metropolitan, urban, rural). The "Basic Geo-Statistical Areas (AGEB) defined by the National Institute of Statistics (INEGI) constituted the primary sampling units (PSUs) and were selected with probability proportional to size"(8). The individual study response rate was 81% (8).

All procedures performed in studies involving human participants were in accordance with the ethical standards of the Research and Ethics Committees of Mexico's National Institute of Public Health and with the 1964 Helsinki declaration and its later amendments or comparable ethical standards. Informed consent was obtained from all individual participants included in the study (8).

Measures

Tobacco use was assessed with the questions, "Have you ever smoked tobacco or used smokeless tobacco?" "Do you currently use (smoke, sniff or chew) any tobacco products such as cigarettes, cigars, pipes, chewing tobacco or snuff?" "In the past, did you ever smoke tobacco or use smokeless tobacco daily?" Responses were grouped into never, past and current (daily or not daily) tobacco use (9).

Sociodemographic variables included educational level, age, sex, residence status and wealth quartiles were calculated based on a 19-item household asset list (using principal component analysis) (10).

Self-rated health status was classified, based on the question "In general, how would you rate your health today?" into poor (bad or very bad), moderate (moderate) and good (good or very good).

Functional ability was measured by the "12-item WHO Disability Assessment Schedule, version 2 (WHODAS-II)" (11), with scores of 25-100 indicating moderate, severe or extreme functional disability (12) (Cronbach alpha 0.90)

Social engagement was measured with nine items on the participation in social activities, e.g., "How often in the last 12 months have you attended any public meeting in which there was discussion of local or school affairs?" Responses ranged from 1=never to 5=daily (13). Scores from the nine questions were summed and classified into three groups of low, moderate and high social engagement. (Cronbach alpha 0.65)

Current alcohol use was assessed with past month consumption of drinks that "contain alcohol (such as beer, wine, spirits, etc.)"

FV consumption was assessed with two questions: "How many servings of fruits do you eat on a typical day?" and "How many servings of vegetables do you eat on a typical day?" Inadequate FV intake was defined as "less than 5 servings of fruits and/or vegetables a day" (14) (Cronbach alpha 0.65)

Hypertension was measured based on the average of two blood pressure measurements and defined as "systolic blood pressure greater than or equal to 140 mmHg and/or diastolic blood pressure greater than or equal to 90 mmHg19 and/or self-reported treatment of hypertension with antihypertensive medication currently (the last two weeks before interview)" (15).

Angina was assessed with the "World Health Organization's Rose angina questionnaire" (16).

Depression was assessed with asking about depression symptoms in the past 12 months using the "World Mental Health Survey version of the Composite International Diagnostic Interview" (17). Additionally, persons who reported to have taken "any medications or other treatment such as attending therapy or counselling sessions for depression during the last 12 months?" were included in the symptom-based depression.

Chronic lung disease and *asthma* were assessed with a symptom-based algorithm (18).

Data analysis

Considering the clustered study design, data analyses were conducted with "STATA software version 15.0 (Stata Corporation, College Station, TX, USA)." Multinomial logistic regression identified predictors of past and current tobacco use (while never tobacco use was the reference category). P values of below 0.05 were accepted as significant and missing values were excluded from the analysis

FINDINGS

The sample included 3,903 older adults (50 years and older), with a median age of 61 years (15 years interquartile range), 55.7% were female and 44.3% male. About one-third of the participants (31.1%) had secondary or more education, 78.8% were residing in urban areas, 29.2% engaged in high social activities, 42.1% rated their health status as good, and 15.6% had a functional disability. More than half of the older adults (56.9%) had hypertension, 11.8% chronic lung disease, 6.4% angina, 4.1% asthma, 11.6% depression, 14.4% consumed alcohol currently, and 85.% consumed insufficient fruit and vegetables. The prevalence of past and current tobacco use was 13.5% and 12.1%, respectively, and among women 7.1% and 6.4% respectively and among men 21.4% and 19.2%, respectively (see Table 1).

Table 1. Sample and tobacco use characteristics among older Mexicans

Variable	Sample	Tobacco use		
		Never	Past	Current
	N (%)	%		%
All	3903	74.5	13.5	12.1
Age in years				
50-59	985 (45.1)	74.8	9.7	15.5
60-69	1424 (29.1)	75.7	14.5	9.8
70+	1494 (25.8)	72.5	18.8	8.7
Gender				
Female	2293 (55.7)	86.4	7.1	6.4
Male	1610 (44.3)	59.4	21.4	19.2
Education				
<Primary	1950 (41.9)	76.2	13.1	10.6
Primary	986 (27.0)	75.5	13.9	10.5
Secondary or more	967 (31.1)	71.1	13.5	15.3
Wealth quartile				
Lowest	954 (21.6)	76.4	12.8	10.8
Low	993 (25.8)	76.0	14.3	9.7
High	1004 (26.2)	74.1	12.4	13.4
Highest	950 (26.4)	71.8	14.2	14.0
Residence				
Rural	1055 (21.2)	82.4	10.6	7.0
Urban	2848 (78.8)	72.3	14.2	13.4
Subjective health status				
Poor	348 (7.9)	78.2	13.5	8.2
Moderate	1898 (50.0)	76.9	12.6	10.6
Good	1657 (42.1)	70.9	14.5	14.6
Functional disability	643 (15.6)	81.8	13.0	5.2
Social engagement				
Low	1418 (38.6)	71.8	13.1	15,1
Moderate	1279 (32.2)	76.7	14.3	9.0
High	1206 (29.2)	75.5	13.0	11.5
Current alcohol use	492 (14.4)	52.1	17.9	29.9
Inadequate fruit and vegetable intake	3293 (85.0)	73.7	13.6	12.7
Chronic lung disease	427 (11.8)	80.0	10.6	9.4
Hypertension	2246 (56.9)	75.5	14.5	10.0
Angina	253 (6.4)	74.8	7.2	18.0
Asthma	157 (4.1)	83.3	8.0	8.7
Depression	442 (11.6)	74.5	13.5	12.1

Associations with past and current tobacco use

Table 2. Associations with past and current tobacco use in older Mexicans

Variable	Past tobacco use	Current tobacco use
	Adjusted Relative Risk Ratios (95% CI)	**Adjusted Relative Risk Ratios (95% CI)**
Age in years		
50-59	1 (Reference)	1 (Reference)
60-69	1.59 (1.04, 2.42)*	0.64 (0.42, 0.97)*
70+	2.26 (1.39, 3.70)***	0.69 (0.44, 1.08)
Gender		
Female	1 (Reference)	1 (Reference)
Male	4.01 (2.90, 5.56)***	3.59 (2.44, 5.26)***
Education		
<Primary	1 (Reference)	1 (Reference)
Primary	1.20 (0.80, 1.80)	0.88 (0.59, 1.32)
Secondary or more	1.09 (9,76, 1.56)	0.81 (0.46, 1.44)
Wealth quartile		
Lowest	1 (Reference)	1 (Reference)
Low	0.94 (0.61, 1.46)	0.70 (0.36, 1.36)
High	0.84 (0.53, 1.32)	0.86 (0.49, 1.49)
Highest	0.89 (0.47, 1.69)	0.82 (0.43, 1.54)
Residence		
Rural	1 (Reference)	1 (Reference)
Urban	1.87 (1.07, 3.27)*	2.62 (1.40, 4.88)**
Subjective health status		
Poor	1 (Reference)	1 (Reference)
Moderate	0.96 (0.54, 1.71)	1.14 (0.60, 2.09)
Good	1.20 (0.64, 2.24)	1.41 (0.74, 2.70)
Functional disability	0.93 (0.58, 1.51)	0.42 (0.25, 0.69)***
Social engagement		
Low	1 (Reference)	1 (Reference)
Moderate	0.90 (0.64, 1.27)	0.56 (0.35, 0.91)*
High	0.98 (0.59, 1.63)	0.67 (0.43, 1.05)
Current alcohol use	1.19 (0.73, 1.94)	2.74 (1.67, 4.50)***
Inadequate fruit and vegetable intake	1.24 (0.80, 1.91)	1.47 (0.82, 2.63)
Chronic lung disease	0.84 (0.49, 1.44)	0.84 (0.47, 1.48)
Hypertension	0.96 (0.69, 1.35)	0.80 (0.56, 1.14)
Angina	0.60 (0.35, 1.02)	2.70 (1.31, 5.59)**
Asthma	0.70 (0.27, 1.79)	1.00 (0.40, 2.49)
Depression	1.08 (0.67, 1.73)	1.04 (0.51, 2.15)

CI = Confidence Interval; ***P < .001; **P < .01; *P < 0.5.

In adjusted multinomial logistic regression analysis, older age, male sex and urban residence were associated with past tobacco use, and younger age (50-59 years), male sex, urban residence, angina, current alcohol use and low social engagement were positively and functional disability negatively associated with current tobacco use (see Table 2).

DISCUSSION

In this nationally representative sample of older adults in Mexico, the prevalence of past and current tobacco use was 13.5% and 12.1%, which seems similar to the global prevalence of tobacco use among older adults (3), but lower than the 2009/2010 Mexico survey (19.9% current tobacco use) (6). As a result of tobacco control policies ("cigarette taxes, smoke-free air laws, mass media campaigns, advertising bans, warning labels, cessation treatment, and youth tobacco access policies"), Mexico has achieved an estimated 30% reduction of smoking rates since 2002 (19). This may explain the reduction of the prevalence of current tobacco use among older adults in this study compared to 2009/2010.

Consistent with previous studies (20, 21), this study showed that with increasing age past tobacco use increased. While current tobacco use only significantly decreased from 50-59 year-olds to 60-69 year-olds, but did not further significantly decrease in the 70 years and older age group. Similar results were also found in a study in South Africa (22). In line with other studies, especially in middle-income countries (6, 21, 23, 24), men were significantly more likely to engage in past and current tobacco use than women, reflecting social and cultural norms (5).

Unlike in some previous studies (20, 21, 23), this study did not find an association between socioeconomic status and past and current tobacco use. Some studies, including in Mexico (6, 21, 23), found a higher prevalence of past and current tobacco use in urban than in rural areas, which was also found in this investigation. Regarding different health risk behaviours, alcohol use was in this study highly significantly associated with current tobacco use, which confirms previous research findings (25,

26). This study found that compared to older adults with low social engagement, older adults with moderate social engagement were less likely to engage in current tobacco use. Similar results were found in a study in New Zealand (27), suggesting that increasing social engagement in older adults may be a way of reducing tobacco use (27).

A previous study among older adults in Indonesia (5) found an association between functional disability and past and current tobacco use, while this study found that functional disability was protective against current tobacco use. While previous investigations found an association between various chronic conditions and tobacco use (20, 24, 28, 29), this study only found an association between angina and current tobacco use. Study limitations include the cross-sectional design, the assessment of some variables, including tobacco use, by self-report, and that certain relevant variables, such as assessing smoking and smokeless tobacco use separately, knowledge on tobacco health, were not assessed.

CONCLUSION

One in four older adults reported past or current tobacco use in Mexico, and several associated factors were identified, such as age, male sex, urban residence, low social engagement, alcohol use and angina, that could assist in programmes promoting the prevention and control of tobacco use in this population.

ACKNOWLEDGMENT

This paper uses data from WHO's Study on Global Ageing and Adult Health (SAGE). SAGE is supported by the US National Institute on Aging through Interagency Agreements OGHA 04034785; YA1323-08-CN-0020; Y1-AG-1005-0) and through research grants R01-AG034479 and R21-AG034263.

References

[1] World Health Organization. Tobacco factsheet, 2019. URL: https://www.who.int/news-room/fact-sheets/detail/tobacco.

[2] Centers for Disease Control and Prevention (CDC) (2018) Smoking and tobacco use: health effects. URL: https://www.cdc.gov/tobacco/basic_information/health_effects/index.htm.

[3] Marinho V, Laks J, Coutinho ES, Blay SL. Tobacco use among the elderly: a systematic review and meta-analysis. Cad Saude Publica 2010;26(12):2213-33.

[4] Bratzler DW, Oehlert WH, Austelle A. Smoking in the elderly: It's never too late to quit. J Okla State Med Assoc 2002;95(3):185-91.

[5] Pengpid S, Peltzer K. Prevalence and predictors of current and former tobacco use among older adults in Indonesia. Asian Pac J Cancer Prev 2019;20(2):395-401.

[6] He W, Muenchrath M, Kowal P. Shades of gray: A cross-country study of health and well-being of the older populations in SAGE countries, 2007-2010. Washington, DC: US Census Bureau, 2012.

[7] Song Y, Zhao L, Palipudi KM, Asma S, Morton J, Talley B, et al. Tracking MPOWER in 14 countries: results from the Global Adult Tobacco Survey, 2008-2010. Glob Health Promot 2016;23(2 Suppl):24-37. doi: 10.1177/1757975913501911.

[8] World Health Organisation. Mexico: Study on Global Ageing and Adult Health, 2014, Wave 2. URL: http://apps.who.int/healthinfo/systems/surveydata/index.php/catalog/212/datafile/F2/?offset=1000&limit=100.

[9] World Health Organization. Guidelines for controlling and monitoring the tobacco epidemic. Geneva, Switzerland: WHO, 1998.

[10] Filmer D, Pritchett LH. Estimating wealth effects without expenditure data—or tears: an application to educational enrollments in states of India. Demography 2001;38(1):115–32.

[11] Ustün T, Kostanjsek N, Chatterji S, Rehm J, eds. Measuring health and disability: manual for WHO Disability Assessment Schedule (WHODAS 2.0). Geneva, Switzerland: WHO, 2010.

[12] World Health Organisation. World report on disability. Malta: WHO, 2011.

[13] Kowal P, Chatterji S, Naidoo N, Biritwum R, Fan W, Lopez Ridaura R, et al. Data resource profile: the World Health Organization study on global ageing and adult health (SAGE). Int J Epidemiol 2012;41(6):1639–49.

[14] World Health Organization. Diet, nutrition, and the prevalence of chronic diseases. Geneva, Switzerland: WHO, 2003.

[15] Chobanian AV, Bakris GL, Black HR, Cushman WC, Green LA, Izzo Jr JL, et al. The seventh report of the joint national committee on prevention, detection, evaluation, and treatment of high blood pressure: the JNC 7 report. JAMA 2003;289(19):2560–71.

[16] Rose GA. The diagnosis of ischaemic heart pain and intermittent claudication in field surveys. Bull World Health Organ 1962;27:645–58.

[17] Kessler RC, Ustün TB. The World Mental Health (WMH) Survey initiative version of the World Health Organization (WHO) composite international diagnostic interview (CIDI). Int J Methods Psychiatr Res 2004;13(2):93–121.

[18] Arokiasamy P, Uttamacharya, Kowal P, Capistrant BD, Gildner TE, Thiele E, et al. Chronic noncommunicable diseases in 6 low- and middle-income countries: findings from wave 1 of the World Health Organization's Study on Global Ageing and Adult Health (SAGE). Am J Epidemiol 2017;185(6):414-28. doi: 10.1093/aje/kww125.

[19] Reynales-Shigematsu LM, Fleischer NL, Thrasher JF, Zhang Y, Meza R, Cummings KM, et al. Effects of tobacco control policies on smoking prevalence and tobacco-attributable deaths in Mexico: the SimSmoke model. Rev Panam Salud Publica 2015;38(4):316-25.

[20] Pang S, Subramaniam M, Abdin E, Lee SP, Chua BY, Shafie SB, et al. Prevalence and predictors of tobacco use in the elderly. Int J Geriatr Psychiatry 2016;31:716-22.

[21] Yawson AE, Baddoo A, Hagan-Seneadza NA, Calys-Tagoe B, Hewlett S, Dako-Gyeke P, et al. Tobacco use in older adults in Ghana: sociodemographic characteristics, health risks and subjective wellbeing. BMC Public Health 2013;13:979. doi: 10.1186/1471-2458-13-979.

[22] van Heerden MS, Grimsrud AT, Seedat S, Myer L, Williams DR, Stein DJ. Patterns of substance use in South Africa: results from the South African Stress and Health study. S Afr Med J 2009;99(5 Pt 2):358-66.

[23] Mini GK, Sarma PS, Thankappan KR. Pattern of tobacco use and its correlates among older adults in India. Asian Pac J Cancer Prev 2014;15:6195-8.

[24] Peltzer K, Phaswana-Mafuya N. Tobacco use and associated factors in older adults in South Africa. J Psychol Afr 2012;22:283–8.

[25] Blazer DG, Wu LT. Patterns of tobacco use and tobacco-related psychiatric morbidity and substance use among middle-aged and older adults in the United States. Aging Ment Health 2012;16:296-304.

[26] Dani JA, Harris RA. Nicotine addiction and comorbidity with alcohol abuse and mental illness. Nat Neurosci 2005;8:1465-70.

[27] Lin EY, Witten K, Casswell S, You RQ. Neighbourhood matters: perceptions of neighbourhood cohesiveness and associations with alcohol, cannabis and tobacco use. Drug Alcohol Rev 2012;31(4):402-12. doi: 10.1111/j.1465-3362.2011.00385.x.

[28] Burns A, Strawbridge JD, Clancy L, Doyle F. Exploring smoking, mental health and smoking-related disease in a nationally representative sample of older adults in Ireland - A retrospective secondary analysis. J Psychosom Res 2017;98:78-86.

[29] Nazir SA, Erbland ML. Chronic obstructive pulmonary disease: an update on diagnosis and management issues in older adults. Drugs Aging 2009;26:813-31.

In: Mexico: Health and Aging
Editors: Supa Pengpid et al.
ISBN: 978-1-53617-950-7

Chapter 6

PREVALENCE AND CORRELATES OF RISKY ALCOHOL USE AMONG A NATIONALLY REPRESENTATIVE SAMPLE OF OLDER ADULTS IN MEXICO

Supa Pengpid*[1,2]*, DrPH and Karl Peltzer*[2,*]*, PhD
[1]ASEAN Institute for Health Development,
Mahidol University, Salaya, Phutthamonthon,
Nakhon Pathom, Thailand
[2]Department of Research Administration and Development,
University of Limpopo, Turfloop, South Africa

ABSTRACT

We aimed to determine the prevalence and correlates of risky alcohol use in older Mexicans. The study is based on a national population-based cross-sectional survey of older adults (50 years and older) (SAGE wave

* Correspondence: Professor Karl Peltzer, Department of Research Administration and Development, University of Limpopo, Turfloop Campus, Private Bag X1106, Sovenga 0727, South Africa. Email: kfpeltzer@gmail.com.

2-2014-15) in Mexico. Self-report using show cards assessed alcohol use. The sample included 3,903 older adults (50 years and older), with a median age of 61 years. Results indicate that the prevalence of risky alcohol use was 3.2%, 6.2% among men and 0.9% among women. In adjusted logistic regression analysis, being 60 to 69 years old and male sex were associated with risky alcohol use. In addition, in unadjusted analyses, higher levels of education, the highest wealth quartile, good self-rated health status were positively and functional disability and depression were negatively associated with risky alcohol use. Almost one in 15 male older adults reported risky alcohol use in Mexico. Several risk factors were identified, which can be targeted in public health interventions.

INTRODUCTION

Worldwide, "harmful alcohol use ranks among the 8th among 79 largest contributors to global disability-adjusted life-years (DALYs)" (1) and is related to more than 60 different types of chronic diseases (2). Risky alcohol use is an established health risk among older adults (3, 4). Studies among older adults in developing countries report a prevalence of risky alcohol use, using different definitions, of 12% in Brazil (60 years and above) (5), 4.0% in South Africa (60 years and older) (6), 13% in Thailand (55 years and older) (7), and about 3.0% in Mexico (50 years and older) in 2009-2010 (8). In a regional study in Yucatán, Mexico, in 2010, 14.9% of participants 70 years and older reported to have three or more drinks per day (9). In the 2001 "National Mexican Health and Aging Study" in persons 65 years and older, the prevalence of alcoholism (measured with the CAGE) was 2.8% (10). There is a lack of more recent national data on the prevalence and correlates on risky alcohol among older adults in Mexico.

As previously reviewed (6), factors associated with risky alcohol use among older adults may include "male sex, younger age, education, income, being divorced, separated, or single better health status, smoking, depressive symptoms and religious involvement." This study aimed to determine the prevalence and correlates of risky alcohol use in older Mexicans who took part in SAGE wave 2 in 2014.

OUR STUDY

The study is based on a national population-based cross-sectional survey of older adults (50 years and older) (SAGE wave 2-2014-15) in Mexico. The dataset is publically available and study procedures and sampling strategy have been described in detail (11). Briefly, a "stratified multistage cluster sampling design" was used to generate a sample that is nationally representative. Strata were defined by locality (metropolitan, urban, rural). The "Basic Geo-Statistical Areas (AGEB) defined by the National Institute of Statistics (INEGI) constituted the primary sampling units (PSUs) and were selected with probability proportional to size"(11). The individual study response rate was 81% (11).

All procedures performed in studies involving human participants were in accordance with the ethical standards of the Research and Ethics Committees of Mexico's National Institute of Public Health and with the 1964 Helsinki declaration and its later amendments or comparable ethical standards. Informed consent was obtained from all individual participants included in the study (11).

Measures

Risky alcohol use was assessed with the question "During the past 7 days, how many drinks of any alcoholic beverage (such as beer, wine, spirits, etc.) did you have each day?" and defined as "the consumption of 4 or more drinks on any day or 8 or more drinks per week for women and 5 or more drinks on any day or 15 or more drinks per week for men" (12).

Sociodemographic variables included educational level, age, sex, marital and residence status and wealth quartiles were calculated based on a 19-item household asset list (using principal component analysis) (13).

Self-rated health status was classified, based on the question "In general, how would you rate your health today?" into poor (bad or very bad), moderate (moderate) and good (good or very good).

Functional ability was measured by the "12-item WHO Disability Assessment Schedule, version 2 (WHODAS-II)" (14), with scores of 25-100 indicating moderate, severe or extreme functional disability (15) (Cronbach alpha 0.90).

Social engagement was measured with nine items on the participation in social activities, e.g., "How often in the last 12 months have you attended any public meeting in which there was discussion of local or school affairs?" Responses ranged from 1 = never to 5 = daily (16). Scores from the nine questions were summed and classified into three groups of low, moderate and high social engagement. (Cronbach alpha 0.65).

Physical activity levels (low, moderate or high) were assessed with the "Global Physical Activity Questionnaire (GPAQ)", it gathers data on three domains of physical activity ("activity at work, travel to and from places, recreational activities") and sedentary behaviour (17).

Hypertension was measured based on the average of two blood pressure measurements and defined as "systolic blood pressure greater than or equal to 140 mmHg and/or diastolic blood pressure greater than or equal to 90 mmHg19 and/or self-reported treatment of hypertension with antihypertensive medication currently (the last two weeks before interview)" (18).

Angina was assessed with the "World Health Organization's Rose angina questionnaire" (19).

Diabetes was assessed by self-reported diagnosis.

Depression was assessed with asking about depression symptoms in the past 12 months using the "World Mental Health Survey version of the Composite International Diagnostic Interview" (20). Additionally, persons who reported to have taken "any medications or other treatment such as attending therapy or counselling sessions for depression during the last 12 months?" were included in the symptom-based depression.

Current tobacco use was assessed with the question, "Do you currently use (smoke, sniff or chew) any tobacco products such as cigarettes, cigars, pipes, chewing tobacco or snuff?" (21)

Anthropometry. Weight and height were measured using standard procedures. Body mass index (BMI) was calculated and obesity defined as ≥30 kg/m^2 (BMI) (22).

Data analysis

Considering the clustered study design, data analyses were conducted with "STATA software version 15.0 (Stata Corporation, College Station, TX, USA)." Unadjusted and adjusted logistic regression was used to calculate predictors of risky alcohol use. P values of below 0.05 were accepted as significant and missing values were excluded from the analysis.

FINDINGS

The sample included 3,903 older adults (50 years and older), with a median age of 61 years (15 years interquartile range), 55.7% were female and 44.3% male. About one-third of the participants (31.1%) had secondary or more education, 66.5% were married or cohabiting, 78.8% were residing in

Table 1. Sample and risky drinking characteristics among older Mexicans

Variable	Sample	Risky drinking
	N (%)	N (%)
All	3903	121 (3.2)
Age in years		
50-59	985 (45.1)	41 (3.2)
60-69	1424 (29.1)	60 (4.8)
70+	1494 (25.8)	20 (1.5)
Gender		
Female	2293 (55.7)	16 (0.9)
Male	1610 (44.3)	105 (6.2)
Marital status		
Single/separated/divorced/widowed	1525 (33.5)	35 (2.5)
Married/cohabitating	2378 (66.5)	86 (3,6)

Table 1. (Continued)

Variable	Sample	Risky drinking
	N (%)	N (%)
Education		
<Primary	1950 (41.9)	43 (1.7)
Primary	986 (27.0)	32 (3.4)
Secondary or more	967 (31.1)	46 (5.1)
Wealth quartile		
Lowest	954 (21.6)	17 (1.6)
Low	993 (25.8)	24 (2.4)
High	1004 (26.2)	35 (3.3)
Highest	950 (26.4)	45 (5.5)
Residence		
Rural	1055 (21.2)	29 (3.0)
Urban	2848 (78.8)	92 (3.3)
Subjective health status		
Poor	348 (7.9)	9 (1.9)
Moderate	1898 (50.0)	44 (2.5)
Good	1657 (42.1)	68 (4.4)
Functional disability	643 (15.6)	4 (0.9)
Social engagement		
Low	1418 (38.6)	40 (3.0)
Moderate	1279 (32.2)	40 (3.7)
High	1206 (29.2)	41 (3.1)
Physical activity		
Low	1966 (46.7)	48 (3.3)
Moderate	1007 (25.4)	34 (3.1)
High	930 (27.9)	39 (3.2)
Angina	253 (6.4)	5 (2.2)
Hypertension	2246 (56.9)	74 (3,8)
Diabetes	944 (23.1)	25 (3.9)
Depression	442 (11.6)	8 (1.5)
Current tobacco use	380 (12.1)	27 (4.7)
Obesity	1132 (35.5)	33 (3.9)

urban areas, 29.2% engaged in high social activities, 42.1% rated their health status as good, 15.6% had a functional disability, and 46.7% were physically inactive. More than half of the older adults (56.9%) had hypertension, 6.4% angina, 23.1% had diabetes, 11.6% depression, 12.1% used currently tobacco and 35.5% were obese. The prevalence of risky alcohol use was 3.2%, 6.2% among men and 0.9% among women (see Table 1).

Associations with risky alcohol use

In adjusted logistic regression analysis, being 60 to 69 years old and male sex were associated with risky alcohol use. In addition, in unadjusted analyses, higher levels of education, the highest wealth quartile, good self-rated health status were positively and functional disability and depression were negatively associated with risky alcohol use (see Table 2).

Table 2. Associations with risky alcohol use in older Mexicans

Variable	Unadjusted Odds Ratios (95% CI)	Adjusted Odds Ratios (95% CI)
Age in years		
50-59	1 (Reference)	1 (Reference)
60-69	1.53 (0.83, 2.82)	1.89 (1.02, 3.49)*
70+	0.46 (0.22, 0.97)*	0.73 (0.33, 1.61)
Gender		
Female	1 (Reference)	1 (Reference)
Male	7.55 (3.99, 14.29)***	6.86 (3.64, 12.92)***
Marital status		
Single/divorced/widowed	1 (Reference)	---
Married/cohabiting	1.47 (0.81, 2.69)	
Education		
<Primary	1 (Reference)	1 (Reference)
Primary	2.03 (1.08, 3.81)*	1.52 (0.78, 2.97)
Secondary or more	3.11 (1.83, 5.27)***	1.70 (0.92, 3.14)
Wealth quartile		
Lowest	1 (Reference)	1 (Reference)
Low	1.52 (0.61, 3.80)	1.60 (0.57, 4.46)
High	2.12 (0.93, 4.80)	1.49 (0.60, 3.70)
Highest	3.65 (1.50, 8.87)**	2.45 (0.83, 7.19)
Residence		
Rural	1 (Reference)	---
Urban	1.12 (0.57, 2.21)	

Table 2. (Continued)

Variable	Unadjusted Odds Ratios (95% CI)	Adjusted Odds Ratios (95% CI)
Subjective health status		
Poor	1 (Reference)	1 (Reference)
Moderate	1.34 (0.60, 3.00)	0.82 (0.34, 1.96)
Good	2.43 (1.06, 5.54)*	1.17 (0.46, 3.01)
Functional disability	0.24 (0.07, 0.83)*	0.39 (0.11, 1.43)
Social engagement		
Low	1 (Reference)	---
Moderate	1.28 (0.64, 2.55)	
High	1.04 (0.53, 2.05)	
Physical activity		
Low	1 (Reference)	---
Moderate	0.93 (0.47, 1.85)	
High	0.97 (0.54, 1.74)	
Angina	0.65 (0.24, 1.77)	---
Hypertension	1.48 (0.79, 2.77)	---
Diabetes	1.30 (0.68, 2.49)	---
Depression	0.41 (0.19, 0.91)*	0.94 (0.20, 4.13)
Tobacco use	1.56 (0.80, 3.07)	---
Obesity	1.24 (0.69, 2.21)	---

CI = Confidence Interval; ***P < .001; **P < .01; *P < 0.5.

DISCUSSION

In this nationally representative sample of older adults in Mexico, the prevalence of risky alcohol use was 3.2%, which seem similar to the 2009-2010 Mexico survey (8), Brazil (5), South Africa (6), and a previous 2001 study in Mexico (10), but lower than in Thailand (7), and a local study in Yucatán, Mexico (9). “Mexico’s alcohol consumption is low by Organisation for Economic Co-operation and Development (OECD) standards – but it is rising, in contrast to most OECD countries” (23), and needs to be tackled by “developing broader approaches to tackle harmful drinking including fiscal and regulatory measures, blood alcohol levels for driving should be lowered to 0.05% in all states, and restrict sales of alcoholic drinks in petrol stations” (23).

Consistent with previous studies (5, 6, 9, 10, 24), this study found the likelihood of risky alcohol use was 6.9 times higher on men than in women. "Biological (sex-related) as well as psycho-socio-cultural (gender-related)" reasons may be responsible for differences in alcohol use (25). Previous studies found that with increasing age, alcohol use decreased (22, 26), while this study found an increase from 50-59 year olds to 60-69 year-olds. This could mean that special attention in alcohol prevention and control should be given to persons in the retiring age group in Mexico. This study found in unadjusted analysis that higher education and higher wealth status were associated with risky alcohol use. Results from former research in Mexico (10, 27) and Brazil (5) confirm a significant association between higher socioeconomic status and risky alcohol use.

Unlike some previous investigations (6, 26, 28, 29), this study did not find an association between single, divorced or separated persons, poor subjective health status, depression, tobacco use and other co-morbid chronic conditions and risk behaviour and risky alcohol use. Study limitations include the cross-sectional design, the assessment of some variables, including alcohol use, by self-report, and that certain relevant variables, such as assessing medication intake, knowledge and attitudes towards alcohol use, were not assessed.

CONCLUSION

Almost one in 15 male older adults reported risky alcohol use in Mexico, and several associated factors were identified, such as age, male sex and the age group of 60-69 year olds, which could assist in programmes promoting the prevention and control of risky alcohol use in this population.

ACKNOWLEDGMENTS

This paper uses data from WHO's Study on Global Ageing and Adult Health (SAGE). SAGE is supported by the US National Institute on Aging through Interagency Agreements OGHA 04034785; YA1323-08-CN-0020; Y1-AG-1005-0) and through research grants R01-AG034479 and R21-AG034263.

REFERENCES

[1] GBD 2015 Risk Factors Collaborators. Global, regional, and national comparative risk assessment of 79 behavioural, environmental and occupational, and metabolic risks or clusters of risks, 1990-2015: A systematic analysis for the Global Burden of Disease Study 2015. Lancet 2016;388(10053):1659-1724. doi: 10.1016/S0140-6736(16)31679-8.

[2] Connor JP, Haber PS, Hall WD. Alcohol use disorders. Lancet 2016;387:988-98.

[3] Blazer DG, Wu L-T. The epidemiology of at-risk and binge drinking among middle-aged and elderly community adults: National survey on drug use and health. Am J Psychiatry 2009;166:1162–9.

[4] Stevenson JS. Alcohol use, misuse, abuse, and dependence in later adulthood. Annu Rev Nurs Res 2005;23:245-80.

[5] Castro-Costa E, Ferri CP, Lima-Costa MF, Zaleski M, Pinsky I, Caetano R, et al. Alcohol consumption in late-life - the first Brazilian National Alcohol Survey (BNAS). Addict Behav 2008; 33(12):1598-601.

[6] Peltzer K, Phaswana-Mafuya N Problem drinking and associated factors in older adults in South Africa. Afr J Psychiatry 2013;16(2):104-9. doi: http://dx.doi.org/10.4314/ajpsy.v16i2.13.

[7] Aekplakorn W, Hogan MC, Tiptaradol S, Wibulpolprasert S, Punyaratabandhu P, Lim SS. Tobacco and hazardous or harmful alcohol use in Thailand: Joint prevalence and associations with socioeconomic factors. Addict Behav 2008;33:503-514

[8] Clausen T, Martinez P, Towers A, Greenfield T, Kowal P. Alcohol consumption at any level increases risk of injury caused by others: Data from the Study on Global AGEing and Adult Health. Subst Abuse 2016;9(Suppl 2):125-32. doi: 10.4137/SART.S23549. eCollection 2015.

[9] Aguila E, Guerrero EG, Vega WA. Sociodemographic characteristics associated with alcohol use among low-income Mexican older adults. Subst Abuse Treat Prev Policy 2016;11(1):16. doi: 10.1186/s13011-016-0061-6.

[10] Aguilar-Navarro SG, Reyes-Guerrero J, Borgues G. Cognitive impairment and alcohol and cigarette consumption in Mexican adults older than 65 years. Salud Publica Mex 2007;49(Suppl 4):S467-74.

[11] World Health Organisation. Mexico: Study on global ageing and adult health, 2014, Wave 2. URL: http://apps.who.int/healthinfo/systems/surveydata/index.php/catalog/212/datafile/F2/?offset=1000&limit=100.

[12] US Department of Health and Human Services and US Department of Agriculture. *2015- 2020 dietary guidelines for Americans,* 2015, appendix alcohol. URL: https://health.gov/our-work/food-nutrition/2015-2020-dietary-guidelines/guidelines/appendix-9/.

[13] Filmer D, Pritchett LH. Estimating wealth effects without expenditure data—or tears: an application to educational enrollments in states of India. Demography 2001;38(1):115–32.

[14] Ustün T, Kostanjsek N, Chatterji S, Rehm J, eds. Measuring health and disability: manual for WHO Disability Assessment Schedule (WHODAS 2.0) Geneva, Switzerland: WHO, 2010.

[15] World Health Organisation. World report on disability. Malta: WHO, 2011.

[16] Kowal P, Chatterji S, Naidoo N, Biritwum R, Fan W, Lopez Ridaura R, et al. Data resource profile: the World Health Organization study on global AGEing and adult health (SAGE). Int J Epidemiol 2012;41(6):1639–49.

[17] Bull FC, Maslin TS, Armstrong T. Global physical activity questionnaire (GPAQ): nine country reliability and validity study. J Phys Act Health 2009;6(6):790–804.

[18] Chobanian AV, Bakris GL, Black HR, Cushman WC, Green LA, Izzo Jr JL, et al. The seventh report of the joint national committee on prevention, detection, evaluation, and treatment of high blood pressure: the JNC 7 report. JAMA 2003;289(19):2560–71

[19] Rose GA. The diagnosis of ischaemic heart pain and intermittent claudication in field surveys. Bull World Health Organ 1962;27:645–58.

[20] Kessler RC, Ustün TB. The World Mental Health (WMH) Survey initiative version of the World Health Organization (WHO) composite international diagnostic interview (CIDI). Int J Methods Psychiatr Res 2004;13(2):93–121.

[21] World Health Organization. Guidelines for controlling and monitoring the tobacco epidemic. Geneva, Switzerland: WHO, 1998.

[22] World Health Organization. The international classification of adult underweight, overweight and obesity according to BMI, 2018. URL: http://apps.who.int/bmi/index.jsp?introPage=intro_3.html.

[23] Organisation for Economic Co-operation and Development (OECD) OECD Health policy overview. Health policy in Mexico, 2016. URL: http://www.oecd.org/mexico/Health-Policy-in-Mexico-February-2016.pdf.

[24] Barnes AJ, Moore AA, Xu H, Ang A, Tallen L, Mirkin M, et al. Prevalence and correlates of at-risk drinking among older adults: The project SHARE study. J Gen Intern Med 2010;25(8):840-6.

[25] Erol A, Karpyak VM. Sex and gender-related differences in alcohol use and its consequences: Contemporary knowledge and future research considerations. Drug Alcohol Depend 2015;156:1-13. doi: 10.1016/j.drugalcdep.2015.08.023.

[26] Merrick EL, Horgan CM, Hodgkin D, Garnick DW, Houghton SF, Panas L, et al. Unhealthy drinking patterns in older adults: prevalence and associated characteristics. J Am Geriatr Soc 2008;56(2):214-23.

[27] Smith KV, Goldman N. Socioeconomic differences in health among older adults in Mexico. Soc Sci Med 2007;65(7):1372-85.

[28] Choi NG, Dinitto DM. Heavy/binge drinking and depressive symptoms in older adults: gender differences. Int J Geriatr Psychiatry 2011;26(8):860-8. doi: 10.1002/gps.2616.

[29] Blay SL, Fillenbaum GG, Andreoli SB, Gastal FL. Correlates of lifetime alcohol misuse among older community residents in Brazil. Int Psychogeriatr 2009;21(2):384-91. doi: 10.1017/S1041610208008326.

In: Mexico: Health and Aging
Editors: Supa Pengpid et al. ISBN: 978-1-53617-950-7

Chapter 7

PREVALENCE AND CORRELATES OF STROKE AMONG A NATIONALLY REPRESENTATIVE POPULATION-BASED SAMPLE OF OLDER ADULTS IN MEXICO

Karl Peltzer[1], PhD and Supa Pengpid[1,2,*], DrPH
[1]Department of Research Administration and Development, University of Limpopo, Turfloop, South Africa and [2]ASEAN Institute for Health Development, Mahidol University, Salaya, Phutthamonthon, Nakhon Pathom, Thailand.

ABSTRACT

This chapter aim to determine the prevalence and correlates of stroke in older Mexicans. The study is based on a national population-based cross-sectional survey of older adults (50 years and older) (SAGE wave 2-2014-15) in Mexico. Self-reported stroke diagnosis was used to assess the

[*] Correspondence: Professor Supa Pengpid, ASEAN Institute for Health Development, Mahidol University, 25/25 Phutthamonthon Road 4, Salaya, Phutthamonton, Nakhon Pathom 73170, Thailand. Email: supaprom@yahoo.com.

stroke prevalence. The sample included 3,903 older adults (50 years and older), with a median age of 61 years. Results indicate that the prevalence of self-reported stroke was 3.1%, 3.6% among men and 2.6% among women. In adjusted logistic regression analysis, high perceived stress, sedentary behaviour and hypertension were positively and inadequate fruit and vegetable intake and low-risk alcohol use were negatively associated with stroke. More than three percent of older adults reported having been diagnosed with stroke in Mexico. Several risk and protective factors were identified, which can be targeted in public health interventions.

INTRODUCTION

Globally, "stroke is the third leading cause of disability and second leading cause of death" (1). In Mexico, according to the National Institute of Statistics and Geography, strokes were the sixth leading cause of death in 2012, just after heart diseases and diabetes mellitus (2). Ezejimofor et al. (3) noted that the "the pooled crude prevalence of stroke survivors was highest in Latin America and Caribbean with 21.2 per 1000." In Mexico, the "prevalence among people aged 60 years or older is 18.2 per 1,000" (4). In population-based surveys among older adults (50 years and older), the prevalence of self-reported stroke "ranged from 2.0% in India to 6.1% in Russia", and 4.3% in Mexico in 2009-2010 (5). There is a lack of more recent national data on the prevalence and correlates of stroke among older adults in Mexico.

As previously reviewed (6), factors associated with stroke may include chronic conditions, such as diabetes, hypertension and obesity, lifestyle factors, such as alcohol use, physical inactivity, smoking, "adding salt at the table", "low green leafy vegetable consumption", and stress, and sociodemographic factors, such as age, sex, wealth status and educational level. This study aimed to determine the prevalence and correlates of stroke in older Mexicans who took part in SAGE wave 2 in 2014.

OUR STUDY

The study is based on a national population-based cross-sectional survey of older adults (50 years and older) (SAGE wave 2-2014-15) in Mexico. The dataset is publically available and study procedures and sampling strategy have been described in detail (7). Briefly, a "stratified multistage cluster sampling design" was used to generate a sample that is nationally representative. Strata were defined by locality (metropolitan, urban, rural). The "Basic Geo-Statistical Areas (AGEB) defined by the National Institute of Statistics (INEGI) constituted the primary sampling units (PSUs) and were selected with probability proportional to size"(7). The individual study response rate was 81% (7).

All procedures performed in studies involving human participants were in accordance with the ethical standards of the Research and Ethics Committees of Mexico's National Institute of Public Health and with the 1964 Helsinki declaration and its later amendments or comparable ethical standards. Informed consent was obtained from all individual participants included in the study (7).

Measures

Stroke was assessed to the affirmative question, "Have you ever been told by a health professional that you have had a stroke?" (6).

Sociodemographic variables included educational level, age, sex, marital and residence status and wealth quartiles were calculated based on a 19-item household asset list (using principal component analysis) (8).

Perceived stress was assessed with two items from the Perceived Stress Scale (9): "How often have you felt that you were unable to control the important things in your life?" and "How often have you found that you could not cope with all the things that you had to do?" Responses ranged from 1 = never to 5 = very often. Summed scores were divided into 2 = low, 3-5 = moderate and 6-10 = high perceived stress (Cronbach alpha 0.87).

Salt intake was assessed with the item, “Do you add salt to food at the table?” Responses ranged from 1 always to 5 never, was dichotomized into often or rarely or sometimes or always = 1 and never = 0.

Fruit and vegetable (FV) consumption was assessed with two questions: “How many servings of fruits do you eat on a typical day?” and “How many servings of vegetables do you eat on a typical day?” Inadequate FV intake was defined as “less than 5 servings of fruits and/or vegetables a day” (10) (Cronbach alpha 0.65).

Physical activity levels (low, moderate or high) were assessed with the “Global Physical Activity Questionnaire (GPAQ)”, it gathers data on three domains of physical activity (“activity at work, travel to and from places, recreational activities”) and sedentary behaviour (11).

Sedentary behaviour was measured with one question by the GPAQ on the “time usually spent sitting or reclining on a typical day”. Eight or more hours a day was classified as sedentary behaviour (12).

High-risk alcohol use was assessed with the question “During the past 7 days, how many drinks of any alcoholic beverage (such as beer, wine, spirits, etc.) did you have each day?” and defined as “the consumption of 4 or more drinks on any day or 8 or more drinks per week for women and 5 or more drinks on any day or 15 or more drinks per week for men” (13). *Current alcohol use* was assessed with past month consumption of drinks that “contain alcohol (such as beer, wine, spirits, etc.)” Responses were classified in no alcohol use in the past month or ever, low-risk alcohol use in the past month and high-risk alcohol use in the past week.

Tobacco use was assessed with the questions, “Have you ever smoked tobacco or used smokeless tobacco?” “Do you currently use (smoke, sniff or chew) any tobacco products such as cigarettes, cigars, pipes, chewing tobacco or snuff?” “In the past, did you ever smoke tobacco or use smokeless tobacco daily?” Responses were grouped into never, past and current (daily or not daily) tobacco use (14).

Hypertension was measured based on the average of two blood pressure measurements and defined as “systolic blood pressure greater than or equal to 140 mmHg and/or diastolic blood pressure greater than or equal to 90 mmHg19 and/or self-reported treatment of hypertension with antihypertensive medication currently (the last two weeks before interview)" (15).

Angina was assessed with the "World Health Organization's Rose angina questionnaire" (16).

Diabetes was assessed by self-reported diagnosis.

Anthropometry. Weight and height were measured using standard procedures. Body mass index (BMI) was calculated and obesity defined as ≥30 kg/m^2 (BMI) (17).

Data analysis

Considering the clustered study design, data analyses were conducted with "STATA software version 15.0 (Stata Corporation, College Station, TX, USA)." Unadjusted and adjusted logistic regression was used to calculate predictors of stroke. P values of below 0.05 were accepted as significant and missing values were excluded from the analysis.

FINDINGS

The sample included 3,903 older adults (50 years and older), with a median age of 61 years (15 years interquartile range), 55.7% were female and 44.3% male. About one-third of the participants (31.1%) had secondary or more education, 66.5% were married or cohabiting, 78.8% were residing in urban areas, 46.7% were physically inactive, 5.9% engaged in sedentary behaviour, 29.8% had high perceived stress, 44.1% added salt to food on the table, and 85.0% ate insufficient fruit and vegetables. More than half of the older adults (56.9%) had hypertension, 6.4% angina, 23.1% had diabetes, 35.0% obesity, 12.1% were currently using tobacco and 11.1% engaged in low-risk alcohol use. The prevalence of self-reported stroke was 3.1%, 3.6% among men and 2.6% among women (see Table 1).

Table 1. Sample and stroke characteristics among older Mexicans

Variable	Sample	Stroke
	N (%)	N (%)
All	3903	127 (3.1)
Age in years		
50-59	985 (45.1)	23 (2.7)
60-69	1424 (29.1)	47 (2.9)
70+	1494 (25.8)	57 3.8)
Gender		
Female	2293 (55.7)	65 (2.6)
Male	1610 (44.3)	62 (3.6)
Marital status		
Single/divorced/widowed	1525 (33.5)	46 (3.4)
Married/cohabiting	2378 (66.5)	81 (2.9)
Education		
<Primary	1950 (41.9)	67 (2.3)
Primary	986 (27.0)	39 (4.3)
Secondary or more	967 (31.1)	21 (2.9)
Wealth quartile		
Lowest	954 (21.6)	28 (2.6)
Low	993 (25.8)	36 (2.6)
High	1004 (26.2)	31 (1.8)
Highest	950 (26.4)	32 (5.2)
Residence		
Rural	1055 (21.2)	30 (2.7)
Urban	2848 (78.8)	97 (3.2)
Perceived stress		
Low	1530 (38.5)	41 (2.3)
Moderate	1268 (31.7)	35 (1.8)
High	1105 (29.8)	51 (5.3)
Add salt to food on the table	1693 (44.1)	48 (2.2)
Inadequate fruit and vegetable intake	3293 (85.0)	103 (2.6)
Physical activity		
Low	1966 (46.7)	73 (3.3)
Moderate	1007 (25.4)	33 (3.7)
High	930 (27.9)	21 (2.1)
Sedentary behaviour (≥8 hours/day)	278 (5.9)	17 (6.9)
Alcohol use		
Not in past month	3411 (85.6)	117 (3.4)
Low risk past month	371 (11.1)	6 (0.5)
High risk past week	121 (3.2)	4 (3.4)
Tobacco use		
Never	2941 (74.5)	85 (3.0)
Past	582 (13.5)	28 (2.7)
Current	380 (12.1)	14 (3.5)
Angina	253 (6.4)	7 (3.2)
Hypertension	2246 (56.9)	94 (4.3)
Diabetes	944 (23.1)	47 (4.6)
Obesity	1132 (35.5)	38 (3.6)

Associations with stroke prevalence

Table 2. Associations with stroke in older Mexicans

Variable	Unadjusted Odds Ratios (95% CI)	Adjusted Odds Ratios (95% CI)
Age in years		
50-59	1 (Reference)	---
60-69	1.05 (0.45, 2.45)	
70+	1.42 (0.57, 3.52)	
Gender		
Female	1 (Reference)	---
Male	1.39 (0.67, 2.89)	
Marital status		
Single/divorced/widowed	1 (Reference)	---
Married/cohabiting	0.86 (0.43, 1.71)	
Education		
<Primary	1 (Reference)	---
Primary	1.88 (0.94, 3.73)	
Secondary or more	1.26 (0.67, 2.39)	
Wealth quartile		
Lowest	1 (Reference)	---
Low	0.99 (0.39, 2.53)	
High	0.67 (0.26, 1.70)	
Highest	2.04 (0.98, 4.25)	
Residence		
Rural	1 (Reference)	---
Urban	1.19 (0.56, 2.51)	
Perceived stress		
Low	1 (Reference)	1 (Reference)
Moderate	0.78 (0.32, 1.89)	0.82 (0.34, 1.97)
High	2.35 (1.02, 5.44)*	2.33 (1.01, 5.39)*
Add salt to food on the table	0.58 (0.33, 1.04)	---
Inadequate fruit and vegetable intake	0.42 (0.22, 0.80)**	0.39 (0.19, 0.79)**
Physical activity		
Low	1 (Reference)	---
Moderate	1.13 (0.54, 2.24)	
High	0.61 (0.32, 1.23)	
Sedentary behaviour (≥8 hours/day)	3.36 (1.40, 8.06)**	3.26 (1.35, 7.86)**
Alcohol use		
Not in past month	1 (Reference)	1 (Reference)
Low risk past month	0.15 (0.05, 0.43)***	0.17 (0.06, 0.48)***
High risk past week	1.00 (0.29, 3.51)	1.03 (0.30, 3.58)
Tobacco use		
Never	1 (Reference)	---
Past	0.90 (0.45, 1.77)	
Current	1.16 (0.36, 3.75)	
Angina	1.04 (0.30, 3.61)	---
Hypertension	2.45 (1.27, 4.70)**	2.24 (1.16, 4.30)*
Diabetes	1.83 (0.93, 3.60)	---
Obesity	1.53 (0.65, 3.69)	---

CI = Confidence Interval; ***P < .001; **P < .01; *P < 0.5.

In adjusted logistic regression analysis, high perceived stress, sedentary behaviour and hypertension were positively and inadequate fruit and vegetable intake and low-risk alcohol use were negatively associated with stroke (see Table 2).

Discussion

In this nationally representative sample of older adults in Mexico, the prevalence of stroke was 3.1%, which is lower than in the 2009-2010 in Mexico (4.3%) (5) and Russia (6.1%) (5) but lower than in India (2.0%) (5) and Ghana (2.6%) (6). Góngora-Rivera (2) proposed, "making massive education campaigns with the information that would permit the population to identify the manifestations of a cerebral-vascular event and permit the urgent transportation to a hospital."

Consistent with previous studies (18, 19) perceived stress was positively associated with stroke. "Stress can increase the cerebrovascular disease risk by modulating symphaticomimetic activity, affecting the blood pressure reactivity, cerebral endothelium, coagulation or heart rhythm" (18). In line with previous research (4, 6, 19, 20), having hypertension increased the odds for stroke. While previous investigations found an association between physical inactivity and stroke (21, 22), this study found an association between sedentary behaviour and stroke. Similar findings were found in a study in China (23).

In agreement with a previous review (24), this investigation found that moderate or low-risk alcohol use was protective against stroke. These "beneficial effects of alcohol consumption have been corroborated by biochemical pathways" (24). In a former review (25), fruit and vegetable intake was protective against stroke and other cardiovascular diseases, while in this study inadequate fruit and vegetable intake was protective against stroke. This finding needs further research.

Unlike some previous investigations (1, 4, 6, 19), this study did not find an association between sociodemographic factors, tobacco use, diabetes and obesity with stroke. Study limitations include the cross-sectional design, the assessment of some variables, including stroke, by self-report, and that certain relevant variables, such as stroke management, were not assessed.

Conclusion

More than three percent of older adults reported having been diagnosed with stroke in Mexico. Several risk factors, such as high perceived stress, hypertension and sedentary behaviour, and several protective factors (low-risk alcohol use and fruit and vegetable intake) were identified, which can be targeted in public health interventions.

Acknowledgment

This paper uses data from WHO's Study on Global Ageing and Adult Health (SAGE). SAGE is supported by the US National Institute on Aging through Interagency Agreements OGHA 04034785; YA1323-08-CN-0020; Y1-AG-1005-0) and through research grants R01-AG034479 and R21-AG034263.

References

[1] Feigin VL, Forouzanfar MH, Krishnamurthi R, Mensah GA, Connor M, Bennett DA, et al. Global Burden of Diseases, Injuries, and Risk Factors Study 2010 (GBD 2010) and the GBD Stroke Experts Group. Global and regional burden of stroke during 1990–2010: findings from the global burden of disease study 2010. Lancet 2014;383(9913):245–54.

[2] Góngora-Rivera F. Perspective on stroke in Mexico. Medicina Universitaria 2015;17(68):184-7.

[3] Ezejimofor MC, Chen YF, Kandala NB, Ezejimofor BC, Ezeabasili AC, Stranges S, et al. Stroke survivors in low- and middle-income countries: A meta-analysis of

prevalence and secular trends. J Neurol Sci 2016;364:68-76. doi: 10.1016/j.jns.2016.03.016.

[4] Marquez-Romero JM, Arauz A, Góngora-Rivera F, Barinagarrementeria F, Cantú C. The burden of stroke in México. Int J Stroke 2015;10(2):251-2. doi: 10.1111/ijs.12189.

[5] Ruan Y, Guo Y, Zheng Y, Huang Z, Sun S, Kowal P, et al. Cardiovascular disease (CVD) and associated risk factors among older adults in six low-and middle-income countries: results from SAGE Wave 1. BMC Public Health 2018;18(1):778. doi: 10.1186/s12889-018-5653-9.

[6] Sanuade OA, Dodoo FN, Koram K, de-Graft Aikins A. Prevalence and correlates of stroke among older adults in Ghana: Evidence from the study on global ageing and adult health (SAGE). PLoS One 2019;14(3):e0212623. doi: 10.1371/journal.pone.0212623. eCollection 2019.

[7] World Health Organisation. Mexico: Study on global ageing and adult health, 2014, Wave 2. URL: http://apps.who.int/healthinfo/systems/surveydata/index.php/catalog/212/datafile/F2/?offset=1000&limit=100.

[8] Filmer D, Pritchett LH. Estimating wealth effects without expenditure data—or tears: an application to educational enrollments in states of India. Demography 2001;38(1):115–32.

[9] Cohen S, Kamarck T, Mermelstein R. A global measure of perceived stress. J Health Soc Behav 1983;24:385–96. doi: 10.2307/2136404.

[10] World Health Organization. Diet, nutrition, and the prevalence of chronic diseases. Geneva, Switzerland: WHO, 2003.

[11] Bull FC, Maslin TS, Armstrong T. Global physical activity questionnaire (GPAQ): nine country reliability and validity study. J Phys Act Health 2009;6(6):790–804.

[12] Chau JY, Grunseit AC, Chey T, Stamatakis E, Brown WJ, Matthews CE, et al. Daily sitting time and all-cause mortality: a meta-analysis. PLoS One 2013;8 (11):e80000.

[13] US Department of Health and Human Services and US Department of Agriculture. 2015- 2020 dietary guidelines for Americans, 2015, appendix alcohol. URL: https://health.gov/our-work/food-nutrition/2015-2020-dietary-guidelines/guidelines/appendix-9/.

[14] World Health Organization. Guidelines for controlling and monitoring the tobacco epidemic. Geneva, Switzerland: WHO, 1998.

[15] Chobanian AV, Bakris GL, Black HR, Cushman WC, Green LA, Izzo Jr JL, et al. The seventh report of the joint national committee on prevention, detection, evaluation, and treatment of high blood pressure: the JNC 7 report. JAMA 2003;289(19):2560–71.

[16] Rose GA. The diagnosis of ischaemic heart pain and intermittent claudication in field surveys. Bull World Health Organ 1962;27:645–58.

[17] World Health Organization. The international classification of adult underweight, overweight and obesity according to BMI, 2018. URL: http://apps.who.int/bmi/index.jsp?introPage=intro_3.html.

[18] Kotlęga D, Gołąb-Janowska M, Masztalewicz M, Ciećwież S, Nowacki P. The emotional stress and risk of ischemic stroke. Neurol Neurochir Pol 2016;50(4):265-70. doi: 10.1016/j.pjnns.2016.03.006.

[19] O'Donnell MJ, Xavier D, Liu L, Zhang H, Chin SL, Rao-Melacini P, et al. Risk factors for ischaemic and intracerebral haemorrhagic stroke in 22 countries (the INTERSTROKE study): A case-control study. Lancet 2010;376(9735):112–23.

[20] Owolabi MO, Sarfo F, Akinyemi R, Gebregziabher M, Akpa O, Akpalu A, et al. Dominant modifiable risk factors for stroke in Ghana and Nigeria (SIREN): a case-control study. Lancet Global Health 2018;6(4):e436–46. https://doi.org/10.1016/S2214-109X(18)30002-0.

[21] Lee CD, Folsom AR, Blair SN. Physical activity and stroke risk: A meta-analysis. Stroke 2003;34(10):2475-81.

[22] Willey JZ, Moon YP, Sacco RL, Greenlee H, Diaz KM, Wright CB, et al. Physical inactivity is a strong risk factor for stroke in the oldest old: Findings from a multi-ethnic population (the Northern Manhattan Study). Int J Stroke 2017;12(2):197-200. doi: 10.1177/1747493016676614.

[23] Yu L, Liang Q, Zhou W, Huang X, Hu L, You C, et al. Sedentary behavior and the risk of cardiac-cerebral vascular diseases in southern China. Medicine 2018;97(44):e12838. doi: 10.1097/MD.0000000000012838.

[24] Rehm J, Roerecke M. Cardiovascular effects of alcohol consumption. Trends Cardiovasc Med 2017;27(8):534-8. doi: 10.1016/j.tcm.2017.06.002.

[25] Aune D, Giovannucci E, Boffetta P, Fadnes LT, Keum N, Norat T, et al. Fruit and vegetable intake and the risk of cardiovascular disease, total cancer and all-cause mortality: A systematic review and dose-response meta-analysis of prospective studies. Int J Epidemiol 2017;46(3):1029-56. doi: 10.1093/ije/dyw319.

In: Mexico: Health and Aging
Editors: Supa Pengpid et al.
ISBN: 978-1-53617-950-7

Chapter 8

PREVALENCE AND CORRELATES OF CATARACT AMONG A NATIONALLY REPRESENTATIVE POPULATION-BASED SAMPLE OF OLDER ADULTS IN MEXICO

Supa Pengpid[1,2], DrPH and Karl Peltzer[2,*], PhD
[1]ASEAN Institute for Health Development, Mahidol University, Salaya, Phutthamonthon, Nakhon Pathom, Thailand
[2]Department of Research Administration and Development, University of Limpopo, Turfloop, South Africa

ABSTRACT

In this chapter we aim to determine the prevalence and correlates of cataract in older Mexicans. The study is based on a national population-based cross-sectional survey of older adults (50 years and older) (SAGE wave 2-2014-15) in Mexico. Self-reported cataract diagnosis in the past

* Correspondence: Professor Karl Peltzer, Department of Research Administration and Development, University of Limpopo, Turfloop Campus, Private Bag X1106, Sovenga 0727, South Africa. Email: kfpeltzer@gmail.com.

five years was used to assess the cataract prevalence. The sample included 3,903 older adults (50 years and older), with a median age of 61 years. Results indicate that the prevalence of self-reported cataract was 12.2%, 12.2% among men and 12.2% among women. In adjusted logistic regression analysis, older age, low physical activity, sedentary behaviour and diabetes were associated with cataract. In addition, in unadjusted analysis, lower education, poor self-rated health status and hypertension were associated with cataract. More than one in ten older adults reported having been diagnosed with cataract in the past five years in Mexico. Several risk factors were identified, which can be targeted in public health interventions.

INTRODUCTION

Age-related cataracts constitute approximately 50% of the 285 million visually-impaired people globally (1). Cataracts are the major cause of blindness and visual impairment in developing countries and contributes to more than 90% of the total disability adjusted life years (2). Based on a systematic review the global age-standardized prevalence of any cataract was 17.2% (3). In a population-based survey among older adults (50 years and older) in six low and middle-income countries (4), the prevalence of self-reported cataract diagnosis was 4.4%, in Ghana 5.4% (5), in South Africa 4.4% (6) and in Taiwan (40 years and older) 11.8% (7). Based on visual disability data from 2010 in Mexico, "65% of the people between 50 and 80 years old will have some form of visual impairment," and from this number 60% could have cataracts (8). In older adults (50 years and older) examined in a "rapid assessment of avoidable blindness (RAAB) in the State of Nuevo León, Mexico," the blindness prevalence was 1.7%, of which 32.6% was caused by cataract (9). There is a lack of more national recent population-based data on the prevalence and correlates of cataract among older adults in Mexico.

As previously reviewed (6), factors associated with cataract may include "older age, lower income, lower education, urban residency, female sex, diabetes, hypertension, obesity, alcohol use, smoking and poor well-being." This study aimed to determine the prevalence and correlates of cataract in older Mexicans who took part in SAGE wave 2 in 2014.

OUR STUDY

The study is based on a national population-based cross-sectional survey of older adults (50 years and older) (SAGE wave 2-2014-15) in Mexico. The dataset is publically available and study procedures and sampling strategy have been described in detail (10). Briefly, a "stratified multistage cluster sampling design" was used to generate a sample that is nationally representative. Strata were defined by locality (metropolitan, urban, rural). The "Basic Geo-Statistical Areas (AGEB) defined by the National Institute of Statistics (INEGI) constituted the primary sampling units (PSUs) and were selected with probability proportional to size" (10). The individual study response rate was 81% (10).

All procedures performed in studies involving human participants were in accordance with the ethical standards of the Research and Ethics Committees of Mexico's National Institute of Public Health and with the 1964 Helsinki declaration and its later amendments or comparable ethical standards. Informed consent was obtained from all individual participants included in the study (10).

Measures

Cataract was based on an affirmative response to the question, "In the last five years, were you diagnosed with a cataract in one or both of your eyes (a cloudiness in the lens of the eye)?"

Sociodemographic variables included educational level, age, sex, residence status and wealth quartiles were calculated based on a 19-item household asset list (using principal component analysis) (11).

Self-rated health status was classified, based on the question "In general, how would you rate your health today?" into poor (bad or very bad), moderate (moderate) and good (good or very good).

Physical activity levels (low, moderate or high) were assessed with the "Global Physical Activity Questionnaire (GPAQ)," it gathers data on three domains of physical activity ("activity at work, travel to and from places, recreational activities") and sedentary behaviour (12).

Sedentary behaviour was measured with one question by the GPAQ on the "time usually spent sitting or reclining on a typical day." Seven or more hours a day was classified as sedentary behaviour (7).

High-risk alcohol use was assessed with the question "During the past 7 days, how many drinks of any alcoholic beverage (such as beer, wine, spirits, etc.) did you have each day?" and defined as "the consumption of 4 or more drinks on any day or 8 or more drinks per week for women and 5 or more drinks on any day or 15 or more drinks per week for men" (13). Current alcohol use was assessed with past month consumption of drinks that "contain alcohol (such as beer, wine, spirits, etc.)" Responses were classified in no alcohol use in the past month or ever, low-risk alcohol use in the past month and high-risk alcohol use in the past week.

Tobacco use was assessed with the questions, "Have you ever smoked tobacco or used smokeless tobacco?" "Do you currently use (smoke, sniff or chew) any tobacco products such as cigarettes, cigars, pipes, chewing tobacco or snuff?" "In the past, did you ever smoke tobacco or use smokeless tobacco daily?" Responses were grouped into never, past and current (daily or not daily) tobacco use (14).

Stroke was assessed to the affirmative question, "Have you ever been told by a health professional that you have had a stroke?" (15).

Hypertension was measured based on the average of two blood pressure measurements and defined as "systolic blood pressure greater than or equal to 140 mmHg and/or diastolic blood pressure greater than or equal to 90 mmHg19 and/or self-reported treatment of hypertension with antihypertensive medication currently (the last two weeks before interview)" (16).

Diabetes was assessed by self-reported diagnosis.

Anthropometry
Weight and height were measured using standard procedures. Body mass index (BMI) was calculated and obesity defined as ≥30 kg/m^2 (BMI) (17).

Depression was assessed with asking about depression symptoms in the past 12 months using the "World Mental Health Survey version of the Composite International Diagnostic Interview" (18). Additionally, persons who reported to have taken "any medications or other treatment such as attending therapy or counselling sessions for depression during the last 12 months?" were included in the symptom-based depression.

Data analysis

Considering the clustered study design, data analyses were conducted with "STATA software version 15.0 (Stata Corporation, College Station, TX, USA)." Unadjusted and adjusted logistic regression was used to calculate predictors of stroke. P values of below 0.05 were accepted as significant and missing values were excluded from the analysis.

FINDINGS

The sample included 3,903 older adults (50 years and older), with a median age of 61 years (15 years interquartile range), 55.7% were female and 44.3% male. About one-third of the participants (31.1%) had secondary or more education, 78.8% were residing in urban areas, 46.7% were physically inactive, 6.7% engaged in sedentary behaviour (7 or more hours/day) and 42.1% rated their health status as good. More than half of the older adults (56.9%) had hypertension, 3.1% stroke, 23.1% had diabetes, 35.0% obesity, 11.6% depression, 12.1% were currently using tobacco and 11.1% engaged in low-risk alcohol use. The prevalence of self-reported cataract was 12.2%, 12.2% among men and 12.2% among women (see Table 1).

Table 1. Sample and cataract characteristics among older Mexicans

Variable	Sample N (%)	Cataract N (%)
All	3903	639 (12.2)
Age in years		
50-59	985 (45.1)	34 (2.9)
60-69	1424 (29.1)	188 (12.4)
70+	1494 (25.8)	417 (28.2)
Gender		
Female	2293 (55.7)	378 (12.2)
Male	1610 (44.3)	261 (12.2)
Education		
<Primary	1950 (41.9)	359 (14.4)
Primary	986 (27.0)	162 (12.0)
Secondary or more	967 (31.1)	118 (9.3)
Wealth quartile		
Lowest	954 (21.6)	152 (11.9)
Low	993 (25.8)	165 (13.7)
High	1004 (26.2)	173 (12.9)
Highest	950 (26.4)	148 (10.1)
Residence		
Rural	1055 (21.2)	142 (9.9)
Urban	2848 (78.8)	497 (12.8)
Self-rated health status		
Poor	348 (7.9)	81 (18.6)
Moderate	1898 (50.0)	320 (12.4)
Good	1657 (42.1)	238 (10.7)
Physical activity		
Low	1966 (46.7)	392 (15.9)
Moderate	1007 (25.4)	142 (11.0)
High	930 (27.9)	105 (7.0)
Sedentary behaviour	310 (6.7)	67 (20.4)
Alcohol use		
Not in past month	3411 (85.6)	566 (12.7)
Low risk past month	371 (11.1)	59 (8.4)
High risk past week	121 (3.2)	14 (10.9)
Tobacco use		
Never	2941 (74.5)	472 (12.2)
Past	582 (13.5)	108 (15.5)
Current	380 (12.1)	59 (8.5)
Stroke	127 (3.1)	616 (16.0)
Hypertension	2246 (56.9)	445 (15.7)
Diabetes	944 (23.1)	204 (18.2)
Obesity	1132 (35.5)	171 (11.9)
Depression	442 (11.6)	97 (15.5)

Associations with stroke prevalence

In adjusted logistic regression analysis, older age, low physical activity, sedentary behaviour and diabetes were associated with cataract. In addition, in unadjusted analysis, lower education, poor self-rated health status and hypertension were associated with cataract (see Table 2).

Table 2. Associations with cataract in older Mexicans

Variable	Unadjusted Odds Ratios (95% CI)	Adjusted Odds Ratios (95% CI)
Age in years		
50-59	1 (Reference)	1 (Reference)
60-69	4.79 (2.58, 8.90)***	4.38 (2.28, 8.41)***
70+	13.30 (7.59, 23.30)***	12.39 (6.82, 22.53)***
Gender		
Female	1 (Reference)	---
Male	1.00 (0.76, 1.32)	
Education		
<Primary	1 (Reference)	1 (Reference)
Primary	0.81 (0.58, 1.13)	1.28 (0.90, 1.82)
Secondary or more	0.61 (0.38, 0.97)*	1.28 (0.82, 2.01)
Wealth quartile		
Lowest	1 (Reference)	---
Low	1.18 (0.87, 1.59)	
High	1.10 (0.74, 1.61)	
Highest	0.83 (0.54, 1.28)	
Residence		
Rural	1 (Reference)	---
Urban	1.34 (0.95, 1.89)	
Self-rated health status		
Poor	1 (Reference)	1 (Reference)
Moderate	0.62 (0.39, 0.98)*	0.75 (0.45, 1.27)
Good	0.52 (0.34, 0.81)**	0.72 (0.45, 1.17)
Physical activity		
Low	1 (Reference)	1 (Reference)
Moderate	0.66 (0.44, 0.98)*	0.78 (0.53, 1.14)
High	0.40 (0.26, 0.62)***	0.62 (0.40, 0.95)*
Sedentary behaviour	3.39 (1.54, 7.48)**	2.20 (1.09, 4.46)*
Alcohol use		
Not in past month	1 (Reference)	---
Low risk past month	0.63 (0.37, 1.08)	
High risk past week	0.84 (0.38, 1.85)	

Table 2. (Continued)

Variable	Unadjusted Odds Ratios (95% CI)	Adjusted Odds Ratios (95% CI)
Tobacco use		
Never	1 (Reference)	---
Past	1.33 (0.89, 1.98)	
Current	0.67 (0.43, 1.06)	
Stroke	1.39 (0.63, 3.06)	---
Hypertension	2.10 (1.52, 2.89)***	1.20 (0.87, 1.66)
Diabetes	1.92 (1.45, 2.54)***	1.82 (1.32, 2.53)***
Obesity	1.03 (0.79, 1.33)	---
Depression	1.38 (0.92, 2.09)	---

CI=Confidence Interval; ***P<.001; **P<.01; *P<0.5.

DISCUSSION

In this nationally representative sample of older adults in Mexico, the prevalence of self-reported cataract was 12.2%, which is was much higher than in other low- or middle-income countries, six countries (4.4%) (4), Ghana (5.4%) (5) and South Africa (4.4%) (6), but was similar to the prevalence in a high-income country, Taiwan (11.8%) (7). In line with previous results (3, 5, 6), this study found a strong association between increasing age and cataract prevalence. Age related cataract is expected to increase with an ageing population in middle income-countries like Mexico (19). Some studies (5, 6, 20) found an association between female sex, lower socioeconomic status, urban residency and cataract prevalence, while this study did not find significant differences. It is possible that different social groups in Mexico have equal access to cataract (screening) services.

A study in Ghana (5) found an association between lower well-being and cataract prevalence, while this study found in unadjusted analysis an association between poor self-rated health status and cataract. In a study in Bangladesh "cataract related visual impairment negatively affected perceived health." (5, 21) In agreement with some previous research findings (7, 22), this study found an association between low physical activity, sedentary behaviour and cataract prevalence. These findings suggest that "maintaining low levels of systemic oxidative stress by being physically active on a regular basis may contribute to the prevention of age-related cataract in the general population" (22).

Having diabetes in this study increased the odds for cataract. Several previous studies have highlighted the link between diabetes and cataract (4-7). Because of the strong link between diabetes and cataract, Pizzol et al. (4) suggest "the introduction of health policies for prevention, early diagnosis, and treatment of diabetes, as well as its complications such as vision diseases."

Unlike previous results (5-7, 20, 23), this study did not find an association between, tobacco use, alcohol use, stroke, hypertension, obesity, depression and cataract. Study limitations include the cross-sectional design, the assessment of some variables, including cataract, by self-report, and future studies should include an objective eye examination.

CONCLUSION

More than one in ten older adults reported having been diagnosed with cataract in the past five years in Mexico. Several risk factors, such as older age, low physical activity, sedentary behaviour and diabetes were identified, which can be targeted in public health interventions.

ACKNOWLEDGMENT

This paper uses data from WHO's Study on Global Ageing and Adult Health (SAGE). SAGE is supported by the US National Institute on Aging through Interagency Agreements OGHA 04034785; YA1323-08-CN-0020; Y1-AG-1005-0) and through research grants R01-AG034479 and R21-AG034263.

REFERENCES

[1] Pascolini D, Mariotti SP. Global estimates of visual impairment: 2010. Br J Ophthalmol 2012;96:614–8.

[2] Rao GN, Khanna R, Payal A. The global burden of cataract. Curr Opin Ophthalmol 2011;22(1):4-9. doi: 10.1097/ICU.0b013e3283414fc8.

[3] Hashemi H, Pakzad R, Yekta A, Aghamirsalim M, Pakbin M, Ramin S, et al. Global and regional prevalence of age-related cataract: a comprehensive systematic review and meta-analysis. Eye 2020. doi: 10.1038/s41433-020-0806-3.

[4] Pizzol D, Veronese N, Quaglio G, Di Gennaro F, Deganello D, Stubbs B, et al. The association between diabetes and cataract among 42,469 community-dwelling adults in six low- and middle-income countries. Diabetes Res Clin Pract 2019;147:102-10. doi: 10.1016/j.diabres.2018.12.001.

[5] Yawson AE, Ackuaku-Dogbe EM, Seneadza NA, Mensah G, Minicuci N, Naidoo N, et al. Self-reported cataracts in older adults in Ghana: Sociodemographic and health related factors. BMC Public Health 2014;14:949. doi: 10.1186/1471-2458-14-949.

[6] Phaswana-Mafuya N, Peltzer K, Crampin A, Ahame E, Sokhela Z. Prevalence of self-reported diagnosed cataract and associated risk factors among elderly South Africans. Int J Environ Res Public Health 2017;14(12):1523. pii: E1523. doi: 10.3390/ijerph14121523.

[7] Shih YH, Chang HY, Lu MI, Hurng BS. Time trend of prevalence of self-reported cataract and its association with prolonged sitting in Taiwan from 2001 and 2013. BMC Ophthalmol 2014;14:128. doi: 10.1186/1471-2415-14-128.

[8] Cruz G R. Epidemiology of cataract in the Mexican population, by 2020. Med Surg Ophthal Res 2017;1(1):MSOR.000505. doi: 10.31031/MSOR.2017.01.000505.

[9] Lopez-Ramos A, Gomez-Bastar PA, Lansingh VC, Rodriguez-Gomez JA, Vargas-Fragoso V, Soria-Arellano FA, et al. Rapid assessment of avoidable blindness: Prevalence of blindness, visual impairment and diabetes in Nuevo Leon, Mexico 2014. Ophthalmic Epidemiol 2018;25(5-6):412-8. doi: 10.1080/09286586.2018.1501498.

[10] World Health Organisation. Mexico: Study on global ageing and adult health, 2014, Wave 2. URL: http://apps.who.int/healthinfo/systems/surveydata/index.php/catalog/212/datafile/F2/?offset=1000&limit=100.

[11] Filmer D, Pritchett LH. Estimating wealth effects without expenditure data—or tears: an application to educational enrollments in states of India. Demography 2001;38(1):115–32.

[12] Bull FC, Maslin TS, Armstrong T. Global physical activity questionnaire (GPAQ): Nine country reliability and validity study. J Phys Act Health 2009;6(6):790–804.

[13] US Department of Health and Human Services and US Department of Agriculture. *2015- 2020 dietary guidelines for americans,* 2015, appendix alcohol. URL:

https://health.gov/our-work/food-nutrition/2015-2020-dietary-guidelines/guidelines/appendix-9/.

[14] World Health Organization. Guidelines for controlling and monitoring the tobacco epidemic. Geneva, Switzerland: WHO, 1998.

[15] Sanuade OA, Dodoo FN, Koram K, de-Graft Aikins A. Prevalence and correlates of stroke among older adults in Ghana: Evidence from the study on global ageing and adult health (SAGE). PLoS One 2019;14(3):e0212623. doi: 10.1371/journal.pone.0212623.

[16] Chobanian AV, Bakris GL, Black HR, Cushman WC, Green LA, Izzo Jr JL, et al. The seventh report of the joint national committee on prevention, detection, evaluation, and treatment of high blood pressure: the JNC 7 report. JAMA 2003;289(19):2560–71.

[17] World Health Organization. The international classification of adult underweight, overweight and obesity according to BMI, 2018. URL: http://apps.who.int/bmi/index.jsp?introPage=intro_3.html.

[18] Kessler RC, Ustün TB. The World Mental Health (WMH) Survey initiative version of the World Health Organization (WHO) composite international diagnostic interview (CIDI). Int J Methods Psychiatr Res 2004;13(2):93–121.

[19] Wang W, Zhang X. Alcohol intake and the risk of age-related cataracts: A meta-analysis of prospective cohort studies. PLoS One 2014;9:e107820.

[20] Rim TH, Kim DW, Kim SE, Kim SS. Factors associated with cataract in Korea: A Community Health survey 2008–2012. Yonsei Med J 2015;56:1663–70.

[21] Polack S, Kuper H, Wadud Z, Fletcher A, Foster A. Quality of life and visual impairment from cataract in Satkhira district, Bangladesh. Br J Ophthalmol 2008;92(8):1026-30. doi: 10.1136/bjo.2007.134791.

[22] Zheng Selin J, Orsini N, Ejdervik Lindblad B, Wolk A. Long-term physical activity and risk of age-related cataract: a population-based prospective study of male and female cohorts. Ophthalmology 2015;122(2):274-80. doi: 10.1016/j.ophtha.2014.08.023.

[23] Bamdad S, Shiraly R. Risk factors associated with cataracts in middle-aged people, an incidence-based case-control study in Shiraz, Iran. Shiraz E-Med J 2019;20(9):e86986. doi: 10.5812/semj.86986.

In: Mexico: Health and Aging
Editors: Supa Pengpid et al.
ISBN: 978-1-53617-950-7

Chapter 9

PREVALENCE AND CORRELATES OF DEPRESSION AMONG A NATIONALLY REPRESENTATIVE POPULATION-BASED SAMPLE OF OLDER ADULTS IN MEXICO

Karl Peltzer[1], PhD and Supa Pengpid[1,2,*], DrPH
[1]Department of Research Administration and Development, University of Limpopo, Turfloop, South Africa
[2]ASEAN Institute for Health Development, Mahidol University, Salaya, Phutthamonthon, Nakhon Pathom, Thailand

ABSTRACT

In this chapter we wanted to determine the prevalence and correlates of depression in older Mexicans. The study is based on a national population-based cross-sectional survey of older adults (50 years and older) (SAGE wave 2-2014-15) in Mexico. The sample included 3,903

* Correspondence: Professor Supa Pengpid, ASEAN Institute for Health Development, Mahidol University, 25/25 Phutthamonthon Road 4, Salaya, Phutthamonton, Nakhon Pathom 73170, Thailand. Email: supaprom@yahoo.com.

older adults (50 years and older), with a median age of 61 years. Depression was assessed with the "World Mental Health Survey version of the Composite International Diagnostic Interview." Results indicate that the prevalence of depression was 11.6%, 6.6% among men and 15.5% among women. In adjusted logistic regression analysis, higher educational level, low physical activity, stroke, and arthritis were associated with depression. In addition, in sex-stratified analysis, angina was associated with depression among men and asthma was associated with depression among women. More than one in ten older adults were diagnosed with depression in Mexico. Several risk factors were identified, which can be targeted in public health interventions.

INTRODUCTION

Late life depression is an important public health problem because of its increased risk of morbidity, increased risk of suicide, decreased physical, cognitive and social functioning, and greater self-neglect (1, 2). The "most common mental disorder among older adults is depression, affecting approximately 7% of the world's older population" (3). In a study in six low- and middle-income countries the prevalence of depression among older adults (50 years and older) was 7.4%, 1.5% in China, 15.2% in India and 10.8% in 2009-2010 in Mexico (4). There is a lack of more national recent population-based data on the prevalence and correlates of depression among older adults in Mexico.

As previously reviewed (5), factors associated with depression among older adults may include "female gender, widowhood, separated/divorced marital status, poor economic status, rural residence, poor dietary habits, lack of physical activity, hypertension, obesity, stroke, cardiovascular disease, arthritis and asthma." This study aimed to determine the prevalence and correlates of depression in older Mexicans who took part in SAGE wave 2 in 2014.

OUR STUDY

The study is based on a national population-based cross-sectional survey of older adults (50 years and older) (SAGE wave 2-2014-15) in Mexico. The dataset is publically available and study procedures and sampling strategy have been described in detail (6). Briefly, a "stratified multistage cluster sampling design" was used to generate a sample that is nationally representative. Strata were defined by locality (metropolitan, urban, rural). The "Basic Geo-Statistical Areas (AGEB) defined by the National Institute of Statistics (INEGI) constituted the primary sampling units (PSUs) and were selected with probability proportional to size" (6). The individual study response rate was 81% (6).

All procedures performed in studies involving human participants were in accordance with the ethical standards of the Research and Ethics Committees of Mexico's National Institute of Public Health and with the 1964 Helsinki declaration and its later amendments or comparable ethical standards. Informed consent was obtained from all individual participants included in the study (6).

Measures

Depression was assessed with asking about depression symptoms in the past 12 months using the "World Mental Health Survey version of the Composite International Diagnostic Interview" (7). Additionally, persons who reported to have taken "any medications or other treatment such as attending therapy or counselling sessions for depression during the last 12 months?" were included in the symptom-based depression.

Sociodemographic variables included educational level, age, sex, marital and residence status and wealth quartiles were calculated based on a 19-item household asset list (using principal component analysis) (8).

Food insecurity was assessed with two questions: "In the last 12 months, how often did you ever eat less than you felt you should because there wasn't enough food?" and "In the last 12 months, were you ever hungry, but didn't eat because you couldn't afford enough food?" (Cronbach alpha 0.88). Responses were grouped into no or low, moderate and high food insecurity.

Childhood health status was measured with the question "In general, how would you rate your health when you were a child, before the age of 10?" (6) Poor childhood health status was defined as moderate, bad or very bad and good childhood health status as good or very good.

Social engagement was measured with nine items on the participation in social activities, e.g., "How often in the last 12 months have you attended any public meeting in which there was discussion of local or school affairs?" Responses ranged from 1=never to 5=daily. Scores from the nine questions were summed and classified into three groups of low, moderate and high social engagement. (Cronbach alpha 0.65).

Physical activity levels (low, moderate or high) were assessed with the "Global Physical Activity Questionnaire (GPAQ)," it gathers data on three domains of physical activity ("activity at work, travel to and from places, recreational activities") (9).

High-risk alcohol use was assessed with the question "During the past 7 days, how many drinks of any alcoholic beverage (such as beer, wine, spirits, etc.) did you have each day?" and defined as "the consumption of 4 or more drinks on any day or 8 or more drinks per week for women and 5 or more drinks on any day or 15 or more drinks per week for men" (10). *Current alcohol use* was assessed with past month consumption of drinks that "contain alcohol (such as beer, wine, spirits, etc.)." Responses were classified in no alcohol use in the past month or ever, low-risk alcohol use in the past month and high-risk alcohol use in the past week.

Tobacco use was assessed with the questions, "Have you ever smoked tobacco or used smokeless tobacco?" "Do you currently use (smoke, sniff or chew) any tobacco products such as cigarettes, cigars, pipes, chewing tobacco or snuff?" "In the past, did you ever smoke tobacco or use smokeless tobacco daily?" Responses were grouped into never, past and current (daily or not daily) tobacco use (11).

Fruit and vegetable consumption was assessed with two questions: "How many servings of fruits do you eat on a typical day?" and "How many servings of vegetables do you eat on a typical day?" Inadequate FV intake was defined as "less than 5 servings of fruits and/or vegetables a day" (12) (Cronbach alpha 0.65).

Stroke was assessed with self-reported diagnosis and/or symptom based algorithm (13).

Angina was assessed with the "World Health Organization's Rose angina questionnaire" (14).

Arthritis and *asthma* were assessed with a symptom-based algorithm (15).

Hypertension was measured based on the average of two blood pressure measurements and defined as "systolic blood pressure greater than or equal to 140 mmHg and/or diastolic blood pressure greater than or equal to 90 mmHg19 and/or self-reported treatment of hypertension with antihypertensive medication currently (the last two weeks before interview)" (16).

Anthropometry

Weight and height were measured using standard procedures. Body mass index (BMI) was calculated and obesity defined as ≥30 kg/m^2 (BMI) (17).

Data analysis

Considering the clustered study design, data analyses were conducted with STATA software version 15.0 (Stata Corporation, College Station, TX, USA). Unadjusted and adjusted logistic regression was used to calculate predictors of depression. P values of below 0.05 were accepted as significant and missing values were excluded from the analysis.

Findings

The sample included 3,903 older adults (50 years and older), with a median age of 61 years (15 years interquartile range), 55.7% were female and

44.3% male. About one-third of the participants (31.1%) had secondary or more education, 6.5% were married or cohabiting, 78.8% were residing in urban areas, 7.% had high food insecurity, 6.8% had poor childhood health status, and 29.2% had high social engagement. Almost half of older adults (46.7%) were physically inactive, 12.1% were currently using tobacco, 11.1% engaged in low-risk alcohol use and 85.5% ate inadequate fruit and vegetables. More than half of the participants (56.9%) had hypertension, 7.5% stroke, 6.4% angina, 35.0% obesity, 14.8% arthritis and 4.1% asthma. The prevalence of depression was 11.6%, 6.6% among men and 15.5% among women (see Table 1).

Table 1. Sample and depression characteristics among older Mexicans

Variable	**Sample**	**Depression**
	N (%)	N (%)
All	3903	442 (11.6)
Age in years		
50-59	985 (45.1)	109 (11.7)
60-69	1424 (29.1)	12.1 (11.8)
70+	1494 (25.8)	161 (11.0)
Gender		
Female	2293 (55.7)	342 (15.5)
Male	1610 (44.3)	100 (6.6)
Education		
<Primary	1950 (41.9)	242 (12.8)
Primary	986 (27.0)	102 (9.8)
Secondary or more	967 (31.1)	98 (11.5)
Marital status		
Single/separated/divorced/widowed	1525 (33.5)	205 (15.1)
Married/cohabitating	2378 (66.5)	237 (9.8)
Wealth quartile		
Lowest	954 (21.6)	85 (11.1)
Low	993 (25.8)	128 (12.3)
High	1004 (26.2)	121 (12.5)
Highest	950 (26.4)	107 (10.3)
Food insecurity		
Low	3127 (79.6)	300 (9.9)
Moderate	535 (13.1)	79 (16.9)
High	241 (7.3)	63 (19.9)

Variable	Sample	Depression
	N (%)	N (%)
Residence		
Rural	1055 (21.2)	83 (6.3)
Urban	2848 (78.8)	359 (13.0)
Childhood health status		
Good	3650 (93.2)	396 (10.8)
Poor	253 (6.8)	46 (22.0)
Social engagement		
Low	1418 (38.6)	190 (14.7)
Medium	1279 (32.2)	123 (9.6)
High	1206 (29.2)	129 (9.5)
Physical activity		
Low	1966 (46.7)	261 (12.7)
Moderate	1007 (25.4)	102 (11.8)
High	930 (27.9)	79 (9.4)
Alcohol use		
Not in past month	3411 (85.6)	402 (12.4)
Low risk past month	371 (11.1)	32 (7.3)
High risk past week	121 (3.2)	8 (5.2)
Tobacco use		
Never	2941 (74.5)	338 (12.4)
Past	582 (13.5)	58 (9.3)
Current	380 (12.1)	46 (9.2)
Inadequate fruit and vegetable intake	3293 (85.0)	385 (12.0)
Stroke	276 (7.5)	65 (32.9)
Angina	253 (6.4)	74 (29.2)
Hypertension	2246 (56.9)	292 (13.1)
Obesity	1132 (35.5)	153 (14.7)
Arthritis	570 (14.8)	113 (23.7)
Asthma	157 (4.1)	47 (36.0)

Associations with depression

In adjusted logistic regression analysis, higher educational level, low physical activity, stroke, and arthritis were associated with depression. In addition, in sex stratified analysis angina was associated with depression among men (OR: 6.11, CI: 1.31, 28.46) and asthma was associated with depression among women (OR: 3.54, CI: 1.34, 7.37) (see Table 2).

Table 2. Associations with depression in older Mexicans

Variable	Unadjusted Odds Ratios (95% CI)	Adjusted Odds Ratios (95% CI)
Age in years		
50-59	1 (Reference)	---
60-69	0.90 (0.48, 1.69)	
70+	0.72 (0.37, 1.40)	
Gender		
Female	1 (Reference)	1 (Reference)
Male	0.40 (0.20, 0.85)*	0.43 (0.19, 1.02)
Education		
<Primary	1 (Reference)	1 (Reference)
Primary	0.94 (0.50, 1.80)	0.95 (0.50, 1.84)
Secondary or more	2.29 (1.22, 4.29)**	2.75 (1.51, 4.99)***
Marital status		
Single/separated/divorced/widowed	1 (Reference)	---
Married/cohabitating	0.78 (0.46, 1.80)	
Wealth quartile		
Lowest	1 (Reference)	---
Low	1.22 (0.42, 3.55)	
High	2.10 (0.59, 6.35)	
Highest	1.84 (0.67, 5.10)	
Food insecurity		
Low	1 (Reference)	---
Moderate	0.78 (0.27, 2.25)	
High	1.23 (0.59, 2.58)	
Residence		
Rural	1 (Reference)	---
Urban	2.14 (0.82, 5.59)	
Childhood health status		
Good	1 (Reference)	1 (Reference)
Poor	2.42 (1.27, 4.61)**	1.90 (0.81, 4.45)
Social engagement		
Low	1 (Reference)	---
Medium	0.57 (0.28, 1.20)	
High	0.86 (0.45, 1.65)	
Physical activity		
Low	1 (Reference)	1 (Reference)
Moderate	1.75 (0.94, 3.23)	1.89 (1.07, 3.35)
High	0.42 (0.19, 0.91)*	0.45 (0.21, 0.95)*
Alcohol use		
Not in past month	1 (Reference)	1 (Reference)
Low risk past month	0.42 (0.18, 0.99)*	0.52 (0.21, 1.30)
High risk past week	0.48 (0.11, 2.03)	0.66 (0.14, 3.20)

Variable	Unadjusted Odds Ratios (95% CI)	Adjusted Odds Ratios (95% CI)
Tobacco use		
Never	1 (Reference)	1 (Reference)
Past	0.93 (0.43, 1.99)	1.28 (0.56, 2.90)
Current	0.37 (0.16, 0.86)*	0.58 (0.24, 1.41)
Inadequate fruit and vegetable intake	0.86 (0.37, 2.01)	---
Stroke	3.58 (1.66, 7.74)***	3.04 (1.37, 6.76)**
Angina	2.56 (1.07, 6.13)*	2.63 (1.00, 6.89)
Hypertension	1.08 (0.58, 2.00)	---
Obesity	1.52 (0.81, 2.86)	---
Arthritis	2.85 (1.44, 5.63)**	2.16 (1.08, 4.31)*
Asthma	2.48 (1.03, 6.00)*	1.86 (0.74, 4.66)

CI=Confidence Interval; ***P<.001; **P<.01; *P<0.5.

Discussion

In this nationally representative sample of older adults in Mexico, the prevalence of depression was 11.6%, which is higher than in the prevalence in six low- and middle-income countries, but similar to the 2009-2010 Mexico survey (10.8%) (4). Consistent with previous studies (4, 18, 19), this study found in unadjusted analysis that female sex was associated with depression. Previous studies (4, 19-22) found a positive association between socioeconomic deprivation, poverty or lower wealth, lower education, widowed, separated or divorced marital status, lower social engagement, rural residence and depression, while this study did not find such associations, only higher educational levels were associated with depression. It is not clear as to why secondary or higher education was not protective against depression, and this finding needs further explorative research. Further, this study found in agreement with previous research (23, 24) that child hood adversity (poor childhood health) increased the odds for depression in unadjusted analysis.

Consistent with previous research (25, 26), the findings of this study showed that physical activity was protective against depression. "A range of biochemical and psychosocial factors are likely responsible, including biological mechanisms" through which exercise reduces depression (26).

This study found in unadjusted analysis that moderate alcohol use was protective against depression, while in a the study among older adults in Spain, "no consistent protective association between moderate alcohol consumption and depression" was found (27). Unlike some previous investigations (4, 28), this study did not find a protective effect of fruit and vegetable consumption on depression.

The study found a strong association between stroke and depression, which has been confirmed in previous studies (29, 30). "Inflammatory processes might be associated with the onset of at least some depressive symptoms. In addition, genetic and epigenetic variations, white matter disease, cerebrovascular deregulation, altered neuroplasticity, and changes in glutamate neurotransmission might be relevant etiological factors."(29) In agreemenr with former research (5, 31, 32), the study found that having arthritis, angina among men and asthma among women were associated with depression. Study limitations include the cross-sectional design and the assessment of some variables by self-report.

Conclusion

More than one in ten older adults were diagnosed with depression in Mexico. Several risk factors, such as higher educational level, low physical activity, stroke, arthritis, angina among men and asthma among women, were identified, which can be targeted in public health interventions.

Acknowledgment

This paper uses data from WHO's Study on Global Ageing and Adult Health (SAGE). SAGE is supported by the US National Institute on Aging through Interagency Agreements OGHA 04034785; YA1323-08-CN-0020; Y1-AG-1005-0) and through research grants R01-AG034479 and R21-AG034263.

References

[1] Blazer DG. Depression in late life: Review and commentary. J Gerontol A Biol Sci Med Sci 2003;58:249–65.

[2] Fiske A, Wetherell JL, Gatz M. Depression in older adults. Annu Rev Clin Psychol 2009;5:363-89. doi: 10.1146/annurev.clinpsy.032408.153621.

[3] World Health Organization. Mental health of older adults, 2017. URL: https://www.who.int/news-room/fact-sheets/detail/mental-health-of-older-adults.

[4] Lotfaliany M, Hoare E, Jacka FN, Kowal P, Berk M, Mohebbi M. Variation in the prevalence of depression and patterns of association, sociodemographic and lifestyle factors in community-dwelling older adults in six low- and middle-income countries. J Affect Disord 2019;251:218-26. doi: 10.1016/j.jad.2019.01.054.

[5] Peltzer K, Phaswana-Mafuya N. Depression and associated factors in older adults in South Africa. Glob Health Action 2013;6:1-9. doi: 10.3402/gha.v6i0.18871.

[6] World Health Organisation. Mexico: Study on global ageing and adult health, 2014, Wave 2. URL: http://apps.who.int/healthinfo/systems/surveydata/index.php/catalog/212/datafile/F2/?offset=1000&limit=100.

[7] Kessler RC, Ustün TB. The World Mental Health (WMH) Survey initiative version of the World Health Organization (WHO) composite international diagnostic interview (CIDI). Int J Methods Psychiatr Res 2004;13(2):93–121.

[8] Filmer D, Pritchett LH. Estimating wealth effects without expenditure data—or tears: an application to educational enrollments in states of India. Demography 2001;38(1):115–32.

[9] Bull FC, Maslin TS, Armstrong T. Global physical activity questionnaire (GPAQ): nine country reliability and validity study. J Phys Act Health 2009;6(6):790–804.

[10] US Department of Health and Human Services and US Department of Agriculture. *2015- 2020 dietary guidelines for Americans,* 2015, appendix alcohol. URL: https://health.gov/our-work/food-nutrition/2015-2020-dietary-guidelines/guidelines/appendix-9/.

[11] World Health Organization. Guidelines for controlling and monitoring the tobacco epidemic. Geneva, Switzerland: WHO, 1998.

[12] World Health Organization. Diet, nutrition, and the prevalence of chronic diseases. Geneva, Switzerland: WHO, 2003.

[13] Pizzol D, Veronese N, Quaglio G, Di Gennaro F, Deganello D, Stubbs B, et al. The association between diabetes and cataract among 42,469 community-dwelling adults in six low- and middle-income countries. Diabetes Res Clin Pract 2019;147:102-10. doi: 10.1016/j.diabres.2018.12.001.

[14] Rose GA. The diagnosis of ischaemic heart pain and intermittent claudication in field surveys. Bull World Health Organ 1962;27:645–58.

[15] Arokiasamy P, Uttamacharya, Kowal P, Capistrant BD, Gildner TE, Thiele E, et al. Chronic noncommunicable diseases in 6 low- and middle-income countries: findings

from wave 1 of the World Health Organization's study on global ageing and adult health (SAGE). Am J Epidemiol 2017;185(6):414-28. https://doi.org/10.1093/aje/kww125.

[16] Chobanian AV, Bakris GL, Black HR, Cushman WC, Green LA, Izzo Jr JL, et al. The seventh report of the joint national committee on prevention, detection, evaluation, and treatment of high blood pressure: the JNC 7 report. JAMA 2003;289(19):2560–71.

[17] World Health Organization. The international classification of adult underweight, overweight and obesity according to BMI, 2018. URL: http://apps.who.int/bmi/index.jsp?introPage=intro_3.html.

[18] García-Peña C, Wagner FA, Sánchez-Garcia S, Juárez-Cedillo T, Espinel-Bermúdez C, García-Gonzalez JJ, et al. Depressive symptoms among older adults in Mexico City. Gen Intern Med 2008;23(12):1973-80. doi: 10.1007/s11606-008-0799-2.

[19] Djernes JK. Prevalence and predictors of depression in populations of elderly: A review. Acta Psychiatr Scand 2006;113:372-87.

[20] Lorant V, Deliège D, Eaton W, Robert A, Philippot P, Ansseau M. Socioeconomic inequalities in depression: a meta-analysis. Am J Epidemiol 2003;157(2):98-112.

[21] Fernández-Niño JA, Manrique-Espinoza BS, Bojorquez-Chapela I, Salinas-Rodríguez A. Income inequality, socioeconomic deprivation and depressive symptoms among older adults in Mexico. PLoS One 2014;9(9):e108127. doi: 10.1371/journal.pone.0108127.

[22] Ortiz ALS, García CIA, Castillo GIA. Determinants associated with chronic and incident depression in Mexican older adults. Gac Med Mex 2017;153(Suppl 2):S102-18. doi: 10.24875/GMM.M17000011.

[23] Peltzer K, Pengpid S. High prevalence of depressive symptoms in a national sample of adults in Indonesia: Childhood adversity, sociodemographic factors and health risk behaviour. Asian J Psychiatr 2018;33:52-9. doi: 10.1016/j.ajp.2018.03.017.

[24] Fryers T, Brugha T. Childhood determinants of adult psychiatric disorder. Clin Pract Epidemiol Ment Health 2013;9:1-50. doi: 10.2174/1745017901309010001.

[25] Stubbs B, Koyanagi A, Schuch FB, Firth J, Rosenbaum S, Veronese N, et al. Physical activity and depression: a large cross-sectional, population-based study across 36 low- and middle-income countries. Acta Psychiatr Scand 2016;134(6):546-56. doi: 10.1111/acps.12654.

[26] Schuch FB, Vancampfort D, Firth J, Rosenbaum S, Ward PB, Silva ES, et al. Physical activity and incident depression: A meta-analysis of prospective cohort studies. Am J Psychiatry 2018;175(7):631-48. doi: 10.1176/appi.ajp.2018.17111194.

[27] García-Esquinas E, Ortolá R, Galán I, Soler-Vila H, Laclaustra M, Rodríguez-Artalejo F. Moderate alcohol drinking is not associated with risk of depression in older adults. Sci Rep 2018;8(1):11512. doi: 10.1038/s41598-018-29985-4.

[28] Saghafian F, Malmir H, Saneei P, Milajerdi A, Larijani B, Esmaillzadeh A. Fruit and vegetable consumption and risk of depression: accumulative evidence from an

updated systematic review and meta-analysis of epidemiological studies. Br J Nutr 2018;119(10):1087-1101. doi: 10.1017/S0007114518000697.

[29] Robinson RG, Jorge RE. Post-stroke depression: A review. Am J Psychiatry 2016;173(3):221-31. doi: 10.1176/appi.ajp.2015.15030363.

[30] Ojagbemi A, Akpa O, Elugbadebo F, Owolabi M, Ovbiagele B. Depression after stroke in sub-Saharan Africa: A systematic review and meta-analysis. Behav Neurol 2017;2017:4160259. doi: 10.1155/2017/4160259.

[31] Wang JK, Su TP, Chou P. Sex differences in prevalence and risk indicators of geriatric depression: The Shih-Pai community-based survey. J Formos Med Assoc 2010;109(5):345-53. doi: 10.1016/S0929-6646(10)60062-9.

[32] Loerbroks A, Herr RM, Subramanian S, Bosch JA. The association of asthma and wheezing with major depressive episodes: An analysis of 245 727 women and men from 57 countries. Int J Epidemiol 2012;41:143644.

In: Mexico: Health and Aging
Editors: Supa Pengpid et al.
ISBN: 978-1-53617-950-7

Chapter 10

PREVALENCE AND CORRELATES OF ANGINA PECTORIS AMONG A NATIONALLY REPRESENTATIVE POPULATION-BASED SAMPLE OF OLDER ADULTS IN MEXICO

Supa Pengpid[1,2], DrPH and Karl Peltzer[2,*], PhD

[1]ASEAN Institute for Health Development,
Mahidol University, Salaya, Phutthamonthon,
Nakhon Pathom, Thailand

[2]Department of Research Administration and Development,
University of Limpopo, Turfloop, South Africa

ABSTRACT

In this chapter we wanted to determine the prevalence and correlates of angina pectoris in older Mexicans. The study is based on a national population-based cross-sectional survey of older adults (50 years and

* Correspondence: Professor Karl Peltzer, Department of Research Administration and Development, University of Limpopo, Turfloop Campus, Private Bag X1106, Sovenga 0727, South Africa. Email: kfpeltzer@gmail.com.

older) (SAGE wave 2-2014-15) in Mexico. Angina pectoris was assessed with the Rose questionnaire. The sample included 3,903 older adults (50 years and older), with a median age of 61 years. Results indicate that the prevalence of angina pectoris was 6.4%, 5.4% among men and 7.2% among women. In adjusted logistic regression analysis, current tobacco use, depression and hypertension were positively, moderate alcohol use, and past tobacco use were negatively associated with angina pectoris. In addition, in unadjusted analysis, perceived stress, edentulism and anxiety were positively and higher educational level and moderate physical activity were negatively associated with angina pectoris. About one in 15 older adults had angina pectoris in Mexico. Several risk and protective factors were identified, which can be targeted in public health interventions.

INTRODUCTION

Angina pectoris is the main manifestation of symptomatic myocardial ischemia and is generally associated with coronary artery disease leading to insufficient blood reaching the heart. Although stable angina is a common initial presentation of coronary disease, and it greatly affects quality of life, work capacity, and costs to society (1). In a large epidemiological study in 31 countries, the angina (assessed with the Rose questionnaire) prevalence was 6.7%, ranging from 0.7 to 14.4% (2). In the "Mexican National Performance Evaluation Survey (NPES) from 2002 to 2003" among adults 35 years and older, "2.3% had a self-reported diagnosis of angina pectoris" (1). In population-based surveys among older adults (50 years and older), the prevalence of angina was 9.9% in China, 9.5% in South Africa and 13.9% in Mexico in 2009-2010 (3). There is a lack of more recent national data on the prevalence and correlates of angina among older adults in Mexico.

Several factors associated with angina pectoris have been identified, including female sex among 55-64 year-olds (2), higher socioeconomic status (1), higher household income in South Africa (3), lower wealth status in China, India and Russia (3), perceived stress (4), depression (5,6), anxiety (7), hypertension (6), diabetes (6), edentulism (1), obesity in Russia (3), physical inactivity (1), low and moderate physical activity in

China (3), smoking in India and South Africa (3). Protective factors associated with angina pectoris may include moderate alcohol use in China (3) and adequate fruit and vegetable intake in Ghana (3). This study aimed to determine the prevalence and correlates of angina pectoris in older Mexicans who took part in SAGE wave 2 in 2014.

OUR STUDY

The study is based on a national population-based cross-sectional survey of older adults (50 years and older) (SAGE wave 2-2014-15) in Mexico. The dataset is publically available and study procedures and sampling strategy have been described in detail (8). Briefly, a "stratified multistage cluster sampling design" was used to generate a sample that is nationally representative. Strata were defined by locality (metropolitan, urban, rural). The "Basic Geo-Statistical Areas (AGEB) defined by the National Institute of Statistics (INEGI) constituted the primary sampling units (PSUs) and were selected with probability proportional to size" (8). The individual study response rate was 81% (8).

All procedures performed in studies involving human participants were in accordance with the ethical standards of the Research and Ethics Committees of Mexico's National Institute of Public Health and with the 1964 Helsinki declaration and its later amendments or comparable ethical standards. Informed consent was obtained from all individual participants included in the study (8).

Measures

Angina was assessed with the "World Health Organization's Rose angina questionnaire" (9).

Sociodemographic variables included educational level, age, sex, marital and residence status and wealth quartiles were calculated based on a 19-item household asset list (using principal component analysis) (10).

Perceived stress was assessed with two items from the Perceived Stress Scale (11): "How often have you felt that you were unable to control the important things in your life?" and "How often have you found that you could not cope with all the things that you had to do?" Responses ranged from 1 = never to 5 = very often. Summed scores were divided into 2 = low, 3-5 = moderate and 6-10 = high perceived stress (Cronbach alpha 0.87).

Salt intake was assessed with the item, "Do you add salt to food at the table?" Responses ranged from 1 always to 5 never, was dichotomized into often or rarely or sometimes or always = 1 and never = 0.

Fruit and vegetable (FV) consumption was assessed with two questions: "How many servings of fruits do you eat on a typical day?" and "How many servings of vegetables do you eat on a typical day?" Inadequate FV intake was defined as "less than 5 servings of fruits and/or vegetables a day" (12) (Cronbach alpha 0.65).

Physical activity levels (low, moderate or high) were assessed with the "Global Physical Activity Questionnaire (GPAQ)," it gathers data on three domains of physical activity ("activity at work, travel to and from places, recreational activities") and sedentary behaviour (13).

High-risk alcohol use was assessed with the question "During the past 7 days, how many drinks of any alcoholic beverage (such as beer, wine, spirits, etc.) did you have each day?" and defined as "the consumption of 4 or more drinks on any day or 8 or more drinks per week for women and 5 or more drinks on any day or 15 or more drinks per week for men" (14). *Current alcohol use* was assessed with past month consumption of drinks that "contain alcohol (such as beer, wine, spirits, etc.)" Responses were classified in no alcohol use in the past month or ever, low-risk alcohol use in the past month and high-risk alcohol use in the past week.

Tobacco use was assessed with the questions, "Have you ever smoked tobacco or used smokeless tobacco?" "Do you currently use (smoke, sniff or chew) any tobacco products such as cigarettes, cigars, pipes, chewing tobacco or snuff?" "In the past, did you ever smoke tobacco or use smokeless tobacco daily?" Responses were grouped into never, past and current (daily or not daily) tobacco use (15).

Edentulism was assessed with the affirmative response to the question, "Have you lost all of your natural teeth?" (16)

Depression was assessed with asking about depression symptoms in the past 12 months using the "World Mental Health Survey version of the Composite International Diagnostic Interview" (17). Additionally, persons who reported to have taken "any medications or other treatment such as attending therapy or counselling sessions for depression during the last 12 months?" were included in the symptom-based depression.

Anxiety was measured with the question: "Overall in the past 30 days, how much of a problem did you have with worry or anxiety?" Anxiety was defined as severe or extreme, as opposed to "none, mild or moderate."

Hypertension was measured based on the average of two blood pressure measurements and defined as "systolic blood pressure greater than or equal to 140 mmHg and/or diastolic blood pressure greater than or equal to 90 mmHg19 and/or self-reported treatment of hypertension with antihypertensive medication currently (the last two weeks before interview)" (18).

Diabetes was assessed by self-reported diagnosis.

Anthropometry. Weight and height were measured using standard procedures. Body mass index (BMI) was calculated and obesity defined as $\geq$30 kg/m^2 (BMI) (19).

Data analysis

Considering the clustered study design, data analyses were conducted with STATA software version 15.0 (Stata Corporation, College Station, TX, USA). Unadjusted and adjusted logistic regression was used to calculate predictors of angina pectoris. P values of below 0.05 were accepted as significant and missing values were excluded from the analysis.

FINDINGS

The sample included 3,903 older adults (50 years and older), with a median age of 61 years (15 years interquartile range), 55.7% were female and 44.3% male. About one-third of the participants (31.1%) had secondary or more education, 66.5% were married or cohabiting, 78.8% were residing in urban areas, 46.7% were physically inactive, 29.8% had high perceived stress, 44.1% added salt to food on the table, and 85.0% ate insufficient fruit and vegetables. More than half of the older adults (56.9%) had hypertension, 23.1% had diabetes, 35.0% obesity, 11.6% depression, 4.9% anxiety, 16.6% edentulism, 12.1% were currently using tobacco and 11.1% engaged in low-risk alcohol use. The prevalence of angina pectoris was 6.4%, 5.4% among men and 7.2% among women (see Table 1).

Table 1. Sample and angina pectoris characteristics among older Mexicans

Variable	Sample	Angina pectoris
	N (%)	N (%)
All	3903	253 (6.4)
Age in years		
50-59	985 (45.1)	57 (5.8)
60-69	1424 (29.1)	84 (5.8)
70+	1494 (25.8)	112 (8.2)
Gender		
Female	2293 (55.7)	154 (7.2)
Male	1610 (44.3)	99 (5.4)
Marital status		
Single/separated/divorced/widowed	1525 (33.5)	94 (6.5)
Married/cohabiting	2378 (66.5)	159 (6.4)
Education		
<Primary	1950 (41.9)	131 (7.2)
Primary	986 (27.0)	72 (7.4)
Secondary or more	967 (31.1)	50 (4.5)
Wealth quartile		
Lowest	954 (21.6)	58 (7.1)
Low	993 (25.8)	70 (7.9)
High	1004 (26.2)	55 (4.6)
Highest	950 (26.4)	68 (6.0)

Variable	Sample	Angina pectoris
	N (%)	N (%)
Perceived stress		
Low	1530 (38.5)	83 (4.8)
Moderate	1268 (31.7)	79 (6.9)
High	1105 (29.8)	91 (7.9)
Add salt to food on the table	1693 (44.1)	113 (7.0)
Inadequate fruit and vegetable intake	3293 (85.0)	219 (6.6)
Physical activity		
Low	1966 (46.7)	144 (7.0)
Moderate	1007 (25.4)	52 (4.0)
High	930 (27.9)	57 (7.6)
Alcohol use		
Not in past month	3411 (85.6)	231 (7.0)
Low risk past month	371 (11.1)	17 (2.2)
High risk past week	121 (3.2)	5 (4.3)
Tobacco use		
Never	2941 (74.5)	187 (6.4)
Past	582 (13.5)	34 (3.4)
Current	380 (12.1)	32 (9.5)
Edentulism	851 (16.6)	70 (9.5)
Depression	442 (11.6)	74 (16.2)
Anxiety	159 (4.9)	19 (16.1)
Hypertension	2246 (56.9)	181 (8.2)
Diabetes	944 (23.1)	77 (7.8)
Obesity	1132 (35.5)	88 (7.9)

Associations with stroke prevalence

In adjusted logistic regression analysis, current tobacco use, depression and hypertension were positively and light or moderate alcohol use and past tobacco use were negatively associated with angina pectoris. In addition, in unadjusted analysis, perceived stress, edentulism and anxiety were positively and higher educational level and moderate physical activity were negatively associated with angina pectoris (see Table 2).

Table 2. Associations with angina pectoris in older Mexicans

Variable	Unadjusted Odds Ratios (95% CI)	Adjusted Odds Ratios (95% CI)
Age in years		
50-59	1 (Reference)	---
60-69	1.01 (0.56, 1.82)	
70+	1.45 (0.85, 2.46)	
Gender		
Female	1 (Reference)	---
Male	0.73 (0.45, 1.17)	
Marital status		
Single/divorced/widowed	1 (Reference)	---
Married/cohabiting	0.98 (0.64, 1.49)	
Education		
<Primary	1 (Reference)	1 (Reference)
Primary	1.04 (0.64, 1.70)	1.20 (0.74, 1.97)
Secondary or more	0.61 (0.37, 0.99)*	0.67 (0.39, 1.12)
Wealth quartile		
Lowest	1 (Reference)	---
Low	1.12 (0.63, 1.96)	
High	0.63 (0.33, 1.21)	
Highest	0.83 (0.46, 1.50)	
Residence		
Rural	1 (Reference)	---
Urban	1.50 (0.84, 2.70)	
Perceived stress		
Low	1 (Reference)	1 (Reference)
Moderate	1.46 (0.85, 2.51)	1.23 (0.71, 2.13)
High	1.69 (1.03, 2.78)*	1.26 (0.75, 2.11)
Add salt to food on the table	1.21 (0.74, 1.98)	---
Inadequate fruit and vegetable intake	1.19 (0.59, 2.37)	---
Physical activity		
Low	1 (Reference)	1 (Reference)
Moderate	0.55 (0.30, 0.99)*	0.61 (0.33, 1.13)
High	1.08 (0.61, 1.92)	1.16 (0.65, 2.07)
Alcohol use		
Not in past month	1 (Reference)	1 (Reference)
Low risk past month	0.30 (0.15, 0.61)***	0.37 (0.17, 0.83)*
High risk past week	0.60 (0.22, 1.63)	0.65 (0.20, 2.11)
Tobacco use		
Never	1 (Reference)	1 (Reference)
Past	0.52 (0.31, 0.85)**	0.56 (0.34, 0.93)*
Current	1.54 (0.80, 2.93)	2.09 (1.18, 3.71)*

Variable	Unadjusted Odds Ratios (95% CI)	Adjusted Odds Ratios (95% CI)
Edentulism	1.71 (1.10, 2.68)*	1.36 (0.85, 2.16)
Depression	3.57 (2.29, 5.58)***	2.85 (1.75, 4.63)***
Anxiety	3.06 (1.48, 6.32)**	1.62 (0.78, 3.34)
Hypertension	1.98 (1.22, 3.23)**	1.86 (1.13, 3.07)*
Diabetes	1.32 (0.84, 2.07)	---
Obesity	1.46 (0.96, 2.21)	---

CI = Confidence Interval; ***P < .001; **P < .01; *P < 0.5.

Discussion

In this nationally representative sample of older adults in Mexico, the prevalence of angina pectoris was 6.4%, which is lower than in the 2009-2010 Mexico survey (13.9%) (3), China (9.9%) (3) and South Africa (9.5%) (3), but similar to a 2002 to 2003 survey in Mexico (2.3% versus 2.0% self-reported diagnosis of angina in this study, analysis not shown) (1). Some previous studies (1-3) found that female sex and socioeconomic status was associated with angina, while results of this study did not show such a relationship. In unadjusted analysis, higher perceived stress increased the odds for angina, which concurs with findings from previous research (4).

Consistent with previous studies (1, 5-7), this study showed that current tobacco use, depression, hypertension and in unadjusted analysis edentulism and anxiety increased the likelihood of angina. The study found that light or moderate alcohol use, past tobacco use and in unadjusted analysis moderate physical activity were protective against angina. These results seem to have been confirmed in previous research (1, 3). Rehm and Roerecke (20) found in their review that "light to moderate drinking has been associated with beneficial effects on ischemic heart disease and ischemic stroke." These "beneficial effects of alcohol consumption have been corroborated by biochemical pathways" (20). In a former review (21), fruit and vegetable intake was protective against stroke and other cardiovascular diseases, while we did not find any association with angina in this study. Study limitations include the cross-sectional design, the assessment of some variables by self-report. Therefore, we cannot conclude a causal relationship between, e.g., depression and angina.

Conclusion

About one in 15 older adults had angina pectoris in Mexico. Several risk factors, such as current tobacco use, depression and hypertension, and several protective factors (moderate alcohol use and past tobacco use) were identified, which can be targeted in public health interventions.

Acknowledgments

This paper uses data from WHO's Study on Global Ageing and Adult Health (SAGE). SAGE is supported by the US National Institute on Aging through Interagency Agreements OGHA 04034785; YA1323-08-CN-0020; Y1-AG-1005-0) and through research grants R01-AG034479 and R21-AG034263.

References

[1] Medina-Solís CE, Pontigo-Loyola AP, Pérez-Campos E, Hernández-Cruz P, Ávila-Burgos L, Kowolik MJ, et al. Association between edentulism and angina pectoris in Mexican adults aged 35 years and older: a multivariate analysis of a population-based survey. J Periodontol 2014;85(3):406-16. doi: 10.1902/jop.2013.130186.

[2] Hemingway H, Langenberg C, Damant J, Frost C, Pyörälä K, Barrett-Connor E. Prevalence of angina in women versus men: a systematic review and meta-analysis of international variations across 31 countries. Circulation 2008;117(12):1526-36. doi: 10.1161/CIRCULATIONAHA.107.720953.

[3] Ruan Y, Guo Y, Zheng Y, Huang Z, Sun S, Kowal P, et al. Cardiovascular disease (CVD) and associated risk factors among older adults in six low-and middle-income countries: results from SAGE Wave 1. BMC Public Health 2018;18(1):778. doi: 10.1186/s12889-018-5653-9.

[4] Nielsen NR, Kristensen TS, Prescott E, Larsen KS, Schnohr P, Grønbaek M. Perceived stress and risk of ischemic heart disease: causation or bias? Epidemiology 2006;17(4):391-7.

[5] Loerbroks A, Bosch JA, Mommersteeg PM, Herr RM, Angerer P, Li J. The association of depression and angina pectoris across 47 countries: findings from the 2002 World Health Survey. Eur J Epidemiol 2014;29(7):507-15. doi: 10.1007/s10654-014-9926-z.

[6] Quashie NT, D'Este C, Agrawal S, Naidoo N, Kowal P. Prevalence of angina and co-morbid conditions among older adults in six low- and middle-income countries: Evidence from SAGE Wave 1. Int J Cardiol 2019;285:140-6. doi: 10.1016/j.ijcard.2019.02.068.

[7] Ketterer MW, Bekkouche NS, Goldberg AD, McMahon RP, Krantz DS. Symptoms of anxiety and depression are correlates of angina pectoris by recent history and an ischemia-positive treadmill test in patients with documented coronary artery disease in the pimi study. Cardiovasc Psychiatry Neurol 2011;2011:134040. doi: 10.1155/2011/134040.

[8] World Health Organisation. Mexico: Study on global ageing and adult health, 2014, Wave 2. URL: http://apps.who.int/healthinfo/systems/surveydata/index.php/catalog/212/datafile/F2/?offset=1000&limit=100.

[9] Rose GA. The diagnosis of ischaemic heart pain and intermittent claudication in field surveys. Bull World Health Organ 1962;27:645–58.

[10] Filmer D, Pritchett LH. Estimating wealth effects without expenditure data—or tears: an application to educational enrollments in states of India. Demography 2001;38(1):115–32.

[11] Cohen S, Kamarck T, Mermelstein R. A global measure of perceived stress. J Health Soc Behav 1983;24:385–96. doi: 10.2307/2136404.

[12] World Health Organization. Diet, nutrition, and the prevalence of chronic diseases. Geneva, Switzerland: WHO, 2003.

[13] Bull FC, Maslin TS, Armstrong T. Global physical activity questionnaire (GPAQ): nine country reliability and validity study. J Phys Act Health 2009;6(6):790–804.

[14] US Department of Health and Human Services and US Department of Agriculture. *2015- 2020 dietary guidelines for Americans,* 2015, appendix alcohol. URL: https://health.gov/our-work/food-nutrition/2015-2020-dietary-guidelines/guidelines/appendix-9/.

[15] World Health Organization. Guidelines for controlling and monitoring the tobacco epidemic. Geneva, Switzerland: WHO, 1998.

[16] Peltzer K, Hewlett S, Yawson AE, Moynihan P, Preet R, Wu F, et al. Prevalence of loss of all teeth (edentulism) and associated factors in older adults in China, Ghana, India, Mexico, Russia and South Africa. Int J Environ Res Public Health 2014;11(11):11308–24. https://doi.org/10.3390/ijerph111111308.

[17] Kessler RC, Ustün TB. The World Mental Health (WMH) Survey initiative version of the World Health Organization (WHO) composite international diagnostic interview (CIDI). Int J Methods Psychiatr Res 2004;13(2):93–121.

[18] Chobanian AV, Bakris GL, Black HR, Cushman WC, Green LA, Izzo Jr JL, et al. The seventh report of the joint national committee on prevention, detection, evaluation, and treatment of high blood pressure: the JNC 7 report. JAMA 2003;289(19):2560–71.

[19] World Health Organization. The international classification of adult underweight, overweight and obesity according to BMI, 2018. URL: http://apps.who.int/bmi/index.jsp?introPage=intro_3.html.

[20] Rehm J, Roerecke M. Cardiovascular effects of alcohol consumption. Trends Cardiovasc Med 2017;27(8):534-8. doi: 10.1016/j.tcm.2017.06.002.

[21] Aune D, Giovannucci E, Boffetta P, Fadnes LT, Keum N, Norat T, et al. Fruit and vegetable intake and the risk of cardiovascular disease, total cancer and all-cause mortality-a systematic review and dose-response meta-analysis of prospective studies. Int J Epidemiol 2017;46(3):1029-56. doi: 10.1093/ije/dyw319.

In: Mexico: Health and Aging
Editors: Supa Pengpid et al.
ISBN: 978-1-53617-950-7

Chapter 11

PREVALENCE AND CORRELATES OF LONELINESS AMONG A NATIONALLY REPRESENTATIVE POPULATION-BASED SAMPLE OF OLDER ADULTS IN MEXICO

Karl Peltzer[1], PhD and Supa Pengpid[1,2,*], DrPH
[1]Department of Research Administration and Development,
University of Limpopo, Turfloop, South Africa
[2]ASEAN Institute for Health Development,
Mahidol University, Salaya, Phutthamonthon,
Nakhon Pathom, Thailand

ABSTRACT

In this chapter we wanted to determine the prevalence and correlates of loneliness in older Mexicans. The study is based on a national population-based cross-sectional survey of older adults (50 years and

* Correspondence: Professor Supa Pengpid, ASEAN Institute for Health Development, Mahidol University, 25/25 Phutthamonthon Road 4, Salaya, Phutthamonton, Nakhon Pathom 73170, Thailand. E-Mail: supaprom@yahoo.com.

older) (SAGE wave 2-2014-15) in Mexico. Loneliness was assessed with one self-reported question. The sample included 3,903 older adults (50 years and older), with a median age of 61 years. Results indicate that the prevalence of loneliness was 12.3%, 10.2% among men and 13.9% among women. In adjusted logistic regression analysis, multimorbidity was positively and being married or cohabiting and higher wealth status were negatively associated with loneliness. In addition, in unadjusted analysis, older age, female sex and functional disability were positively and moderate or high physical activity, light or moderate alcohol use and higher educational levels were negatively associated with loneliness. More than one in ten older adults in Mexico reported loneliness. Several risk and protective factors were identified, which can be targeted in public health interventions.

INTRODUCTION

Loneliness is a "distressing feeling that accompanies the perception that one's social needs are not being met by the quantity or especially the quality of one's social relationships" (1) and may be a "common phenomenon in old age due to changes in the quality and quantity of social relationships" (2, 3). "Loneliness and isolation have a detrimental effect on health in old age" (4). The prevalence of loneliness among older adults in 11 European countries has been found to be common, ranging from 10% in France and Norway to more than 30% in Bulgaria (5). In a middle-income country, South Africa, the prevalence of self-reported loneliness was among older adults 9.9% (6), almost 10% of 70 to 74 year-olds in Indonesia reported occasionally or all of the time to be lonely (7), and in Malaysia about "one third of older adults reported a lot of loneliness" (8). In a population-based study of the "Coyoacán Cohort aged 70 and older" (N = 927) in Mexico, the prevalence of loneliness was 13.2% (based on the "Short Form of the Revised University of California at Los Angeles Loneliness Scale score ≥ 6") (9). In a qualitative study among persons 60 years and older residing in rural areas (Guerrero and Morelos) in Mexico, "the main fears associated with aging are loneliness, illness, poverty, and loss of independence" (10). There is a lack of more recent national data on the prevalence and correlates of loneliness among older adults in Mexico (11, 12).

Several risk factors associated with loneliness have been identified (7, 13), including sex, age, lower socioeconomic status and adverse childhood experiences and several protective factors include social support, being married, social capital (high levels of trust) and social engagement. This study aimed to determine the prevalence and correlates of loneliness in older Mexicans who took part in SAGE wave 2 in 2014.

OUR STUDY

The study is based on a national population-based cross-sectional survey of older adults (50 years and older) (SAGE wave 2-2014-15) in Mexico. The dataset is publically available and study procedures and sampling strategy have been described in detail (14). Briefly, a "stratified multistage cluster sampling design" was used to generate a sample that is nationally representative. Strata were defined by locality (metropolitan, urban, rural). The "Basic Geo-Statistical Areas (AGEB) defined by the National Institute of Statistics (INEGI) constituted the primary sampling units (PSUs) and were selected with probability proportional to size" (14). The individual study response rate was 81% (14).

All procedures performed in studies involving human participants were in accordance with the ethical standards of the Research and Ethics Committees of Mexico's National Institute of Public Health and with the 1964 Helsinki declaration and its later amendments or comparable ethical standards. Informed consent was obtained from all individual participants included in the study (14).

Measures

Loneliness was defined as affirmative response to the question "Did you feel lonely for much of the day yesterday?"

Sociodemographic variables included educational level, age, sex, marital and residence status and wealth quartiles were calculated based on a 19-item household asset list (using principal component analysis) (15).

Social engagement was measured with nine items on the participation in social activities, e.g., "How often in the last 12 months have you attended any public meeting in which there was discussion of local or school affairs?" Responses ranged from 1 = never to 5 = daily. Scores from the nine questions were summed and classified into three groups of low, moderate and high social engagement (Cronbach alpha 0.65).

Trust was measured with five questions, e.g., "Generally speaking, would you say that most people can be trusted or that you can't be too careful in dealing with people?" Scores from the five questions were summed and grouped into low, median and high trust (16) (Cronbach alpha 0.65).

Unsafe environment was assessed with two items, e.g., "In general, how safe from crime and violence do you feel when you are alone at home?" Scores from the two questions were summed and classified into three groups of low, moderate and high unsafe environment (16) (Cronbach alpha 0.66).

Childhood health status was measured with the question "In general, how would you rate your health when you were a child, before the age of 10?" Poor childhood health status was defined as moderate, bad or very bad and good childhood health status as good or very good.

Physical activity levels (low, moderate or high) were assessed with the "Global Physical Activity Questionnaire (GPAQ)," it gathers data on three domains of physical activity ("activity at work, travel to and from places, recreational activities") and sedentary behaviour (17).

High-risk alcohol use was assessed with the question "During the past 7 days, how many drinks of any alcoholic beverage (such as beer, wine, spirits, etc.) did you have each day?" and defined as "the consumption of 4 or more drinks on any day or 8 or more drinks per week for women and 5 or more drinks on any day or 15 or more drinks per week for men" (18). *Current alcohol use* was assessed with past month consumption of drinks that "contain alcohol (such as beer, wine, spirits, etc.)" Responses were classified in no alcohol use in the past month or ever, low-risk alcohol use in the past month and high-risk alcohol use in the past week.

Tobacco use was assessed with the questions, "Have you ever smoked tobacco or used smokeless tobacco?" "Do you currently use (smoke, sniff or chew) any tobacco products such as cigarettes, cigars, pipes, chewing tobacco or snuff?" "In the past, did you ever smoke tobacco or use smokeless tobacco daily?" Responses were grouped into never, past and current (daily or not daily) tobacco use (19).

Multimorbidity was defined as "two or more chronic physical health conditions (angina, arthritis, asthma, chronic back pain, chronic lung disease, diabetes, edentulism, hearing problems, hypertension, stroke, visual impairment)" (20). *Angina* was assessed with the "World Health Organization's Rose angina questionnaire" (21). *Chronic back pain* was defined as "having had back pain every day during the last 30 days." (20). *Edentulism* was assessed with the affirmative response to the question, "Have you lost all of your natural teeth?" (22). *Diabetes and stroke* were assessed by self-reported diagnosis. *Hearing problems* was accepted if "the interviewer observed this condition during the survey."(20) *Visual impairment* was defined as "having severe or extreme difficulty in seeing and recognizing a person that the participant knows across the road." *Hypertension* was measured based on the average of two blood pressure measurements and defined as "systolic blood pressure greater than or equal to 140 mmHg and/or diastolic blood pressure greater than or equal to 90 mmHg19 and/or self-reported treatment of hypertension with antihypertensive medication currently (the last two weeks before interview)" (23). *Arthritis, asthma and chronic lung disease* were assessed with a symptom-based algorithm (24).

Functional ability was measured by the "12-item WHO Disability Assessment Schedule, version 2 (WHODAS-II)" (25), with scores of 25-100 indicating moderate, severe or extreme functional disability (26) (Cronbach alpha 0.90).

Data analysis

Considering the clustered study design, data analyses were conducted with STATA software version 15.0 (Stata Corporation, College Station, TX, USA). Unadjusted and adjusted logistic regression was used to calculate predictors of loneliness. P values of below 0.05 were accepted as significant and missing values were excluded from the analysis.

FINDINGS

The sample included 3,903 older adults (50 years and older), with a median age of 61 years (15 years interquartile range), 55.7% were female and 44.3% male. About one-third of the participants (31.1%) had secondary or more education, 66.5% were married or cohabiting, 78.8% were residing in urban areas, 46.7% were physically inactive, 29.2% had high social engagement, 29.6% high trust, and 40.9% a highly unsafe environment. Almost half of the older adults (45.9%) had two or more physical chronic conditions, 15.6% had a functional disability, 12.1% were currently using tobacco and 11.1% engaged in low-risk alcohol use. The prevalence of loneliness was 12.3%, 10.2% among men and 13.9% among women (see Table 1).

Table 1. Sample and loneliness characteristics among older Mexicans

Variable	Sample	Loneliness
	N (%)	N (%)
All	3903	558 (12.3)
Age in years		
50-59	985 (45.1)	102 (9.6)
60-69	1424 (29.1)	186 (11.6)
70+	1494 (25.8)	270 (17.7)
Gender		
Female	2293 (55.7)	352 (13.9)
Male	1610 (44.3)	206 (10.2)

Variable	Sample	Loneliness
	N (%)	N (%)
Marital status		
Single/separated/divorced/widowed	1525 (33.5)	302 (19.0)
Married/cohabiting	2378 (66.5)	256 (8.9)
Education		
<Primary	1950 (41.9)	362 (16.5)
Primary	986 (27.0)	116 (10.1)
Secondary or more	967 (31.1)	80 (8.4)
Wealth quartile		
Lowest	954 (21.6)	198 (17.8)
Low	993 (25.8)	167 (15.1)
High	1004 (26.2)	115 (9.4)
Highest	950 (26.4)	77 (7.7)
Residence		
Rural	1055 (21.2)	178 (14.5)
Urban	2848 (78.8)	380 (11.7)
Social engagement		
Low	1418 (38.6)	235 (13.3)
Moderate	1279 (32.2)	170 (11.8)
High	1206 (29.2)	153 (11.4)
Trust		
Low	1361 (37.0)	217 (14.8)
Medium	1320 (33.4)	177 (10.3)
High	1222 (29.6)	164 (11.2)
Unsafe environment		
Low	1248 (30.0)	163 (11.4)
Moderate	1227 (29.2)	173 (11.7)
High	1428 (40.9)	222 (13.4)
Childhood health status		
Good	3650 (93.2)	515 (11.8)
Poor	253 (6.8)	43 (18.2)
Physical activity		
Low	1966 (46.7)	328 (15.1)
Moderate	1007 (25.4)	125 (10.2)
High	930 (27.9)	105 (9.4)
Alcohol use		
Not in past month	3411 (85.6)	505 (13.1)
Low risk past month	371 (11.1)	36 (5.8)
High risk past week	121 (3.2)	17 (12.7)
Tobacco use		
Never	2941 (74.5)	422 (12.6)
Past	582 (13.5)	76 (10.9)
Current	380 (12.1)	60 (12.0)
Multimorbidity	1840 (45.9)	336 (17.3)
Functional disability	643 (15.6)	167 (22.6)

Associations with loneliness

In adjusted logistic regression analysis, multimorbidity was positively and being married or cohabiting and higher wealth status were negatively associated with loneliness. In addition, in unadjusted analysis, older age, female sex and functional disability were positively and moderate or high physical activity, light or moderate alcohol use and higher educational levels were negatively associated with loneliness (see Table 2).

Table 2. Associations with loneliness in older Mexicans

Variable	Unadjusted Odds Ratios (95% CI)	Adjusted Odds Ratios (95% CI)
Age in years		
50-59	1 (Reference)	1 (Reference)
60-69	1.23 (0.83, 1.83)	1.01 (0.64, 1.58)
70+	2.02 (1.33, 3.07)***	1.00 (0.61, 1.63)
Gender		
Female	1 (Reference)	1 (Reference)
Male	0.71 (0.52, 0.96)*	0.99 (0.69, 1.40)
Marital status		
Single/separated/divorced/widowed	1 (Reference)	1 (Reference)
Married/cohabiting	0.42 (0.31, 0.56)***	0.47 (0.32, 0.70)***
Education		
<Primary	1 (Reference)	1 (Reference)
Primary	0.57 (0.42, 0.77)***	0.70 (0.48, 1.03)
Secondary or more	0.47 (0.31, 0.70)***	0.70 (0.45, 1.08)
Wealth quartile		
Lowest	1 (Reference)	1 (Reference)
Low	0.82 (0.62, 1.08)	0.92 (0.66, 1.26)
High	0.48 (0.31, 0.75)**	0.59 (0.37, 0.93)*
Highest	0.38 (0.24, 0.61)***	0.56 (0.32, 0.97)*
Residence		
Rural	1 (Reference)	---
Urban	0.78 (0.58, 1.06)	
Social engagement		
Low	1 (Reference)	---
Moderate	0.88 (0.64, 1.21)	
High	0.83 (0.58, 1.22)	

Variable	Unadjusted Odds Ratios (95% CI)	Adjusted Odds Ratios (95% CI)
Trust		
Low	1 (Reference)	---
Medium	0.66 (0.45, 0.98)	
High	0.72 (0.51, 1.03)	
Unsafe environment		
Low	1 (Reference)	---
Moderate	1.03 (0.70, 1.52)	
High	1.20 (0.79, 1.82)	
Childhood health status		
Good	1 (Reference)	---
Poor	1.66 (0.97, 2.81)	
Physical activity		
Low	1 (Reference)	1 (Reference)
Moderate	0.64 (0.42, 0.97)*	0.73 (0.45, 1.18)
High	0.58 (0.40, 0.85)***	0.78 (0.51, 1.19)
Alcohol use		
Not in past month	1 (Reference)	1 (Reference)
Low risk past month	0.41 (0.22, 0.76)**	0.76 (0.41, 1.41)
High risk past week	0.97 (0.47, 2.01)	1.49 (0.65, 3.44)
Tobacco use		
Never	1 (Reference)	---
Past	0.85 (0.56, 1.29)	
Current	0.95 (0.56, 1.60)	
Multimorbidity	2.30 (1.73, 3.06)***	1.85 (1.29, 3.65)***
Functional disability	2.46 (1.68, 3.60)***	1.58 (0.96, 2.61)

CI = Confidence Interval; ***P < .001; **P < .01; *P < 0.5.

DISCUSSION

In this nationally representative sample of older adults in Mexico, the prevalence of loneliness was 12.3%, which is higher than in a number of European countries (5), South Africa (6) and Indonesia (7). Among person 70 years and older the prevalence of loneliness was in this study 17.7%, which is higher than in a previous local study in rural Mexico (13.2%) (9). "Promising interventions targeting loneliness and social isolation among older adults may include new technologies and community engaged arts" (27).

This study found that lower wealth status and in unadjusted analysis lower education, female sex and older age were associated with loneliness. These results are consistent with previous research findings (6, 7, 13). It is possible that older adults with lower wealth status "have less resources and opportunities that could prevent them becoming lonely" (13). Unlike some previous studies (7, 28), this study did not find an association between rural residence, childhood adversity (poor health status) and loneliness.

In line with previous results (6, 7, 13) being separated, divorced, widowed or never married increased the odds for loneliness signicifantly in this study. Unlike previous research (7, 29, 30), this study did not find any association between measures of social capital (social engagement, trust and safe environment). Having multiple chronic conditions and in unadjusted analysis functional disability were in this study associated with loneliness. These results were found previously (6, 7) and "may be explained by the limiting effect of having chronic conditions and/or having functional disability on the participation and performance of specifc activities" (6, 7, 31).

Some investigations (30, 32-34) found that certain health risk behaviours, such as tobacco use, physical inactivity and alcohol use, were higher in individuals with loneliness compared to those who were not lonely, while this study found in unadjusted analysis that moderate and high physical activity and light or moderate alcohol use were protective from loneliness. Study limitations include the cross-sectional design, the assessment of some variables by self-report and loneliness was only assessed with one item. However, some research seem to indicate "a high correlation between single-item and multi-item loneliness indices." (35) Some question, e.g., on living status (living alone, etc.), were not included in this study and should be incorporated in futher investigations.

CONCLUSION

More than one in ten older adults in Mexico reported loneliness. Several risk factors, such as multimorbidity and in unadjusted analysis older age, female sex and functional disability, and several protective factors (being married or cohabiting and higher wealth status and in unadjusted analysis moderate or high physical activity, light or moderate alcohol use and higher educationl levels) were identified, which can be targeted in public health interventions.

ACKNOWLEDGMENTS

This paper uses data from WHO's Study on Global Ageing and Adult Health (SAGE). SAGE is supported by the US National Institute on Aging through Interagency Agreements OGHA 04034785; YA1323-08-CN-0020; Y1-AG-1005-0) and through research grants R01-AG034479 and R21-AG034263.

REFERENCES

[1] Hawkley LC, Cacioppo JT. Loneliness matters: a theoretical and empirical review of consequences and mechanisms. Ann Behav Med 2010;40:218-27. https://doi.org/10.1007/s12160-010-9210-8.

[2] Qualter P, Vanhalst J, Harris R, Van Roekel E, Lodder G, Bangee M, et al. Loneliness across the life span. Perspect Psychol Sci 2015;10:250-64.

[3] Luanaigh CO, Lawlor BA. Loneliness and the health of older people. Int J Geriatric Psychiatry 2008:23(12):1213-21. doi: 10.1002/gps.2054.

[4] Courtin E, Knapp M. Social isolation, loneliness and health in old age: a scoping review. Health Soc Care Community 2017;25(3):799-812. doi: 10.1111/hsc.12311.

[5] Hansen T, Slagsvold B. Late-life loneliness in 11 European countries: Results from the generations and gender survey. Soc Indic Res 2016;129:445-64. doi:10.1007/s11205-015-1111-6.

[6] Phaswana-Mafuya N, Peltzer K. Loneliness and health among older adults in South Africa. Glob J Health Sci 2017;9(12):1. doi:10.5539/gjhs.v9n12p1.

[7] Peltzer K, Pengpid S. Loneliness correlates and associations with health variables in the general population in Indonesia. Int J Ment Health Syst 2019;13:24. https://doi.org/10.1186/s13033-019-0281-z.

[8] Momtaz YA, Hamid TA, Yusof S, Ibrahim R, Chai ST, Yahaya N, Abdullah SS. Loneliness as a risk factor for hypertension in later life. J Aging Health 2012;24(4):696–710. https://doi.org/10.1177/0898264311431305.

[9] Herrera-Badilla A, Navarrete-Reyes AP, Amieva H, Avila-Funes JA. Loneliness is associated with frailty in community-dwelling elderly adults. J Am Geriatr Soc 2015;63(3):607-9. doi: 10.1111/jgs.13308.

[10] Treviño-Siller S, Pelcastre-Villafuerte B, Márquez-Serrano M. Aging experiences in rural Mexico. Salud Publica Mex 2006;48(1):30-8.

[11] Montero-López Lena M, Luna-Bazaldúa D, Shneidman LA. Loneliness in the elderly in Mexico, challenges to the public policies. J Chin Sociol 2019;6:16. https://doi.org/10.1186/s40711-019-0106-0.

[12] Ortiz ALS, García CIA, Castillo GIA. Determinants associated with chronic and incident depression in Mexican older adults. Gac Med Mex 2017;153(Suppl 2):S102-18. doi: 10.24875/GMM.M17000011.

[13] Cohen-Mansfield J, Hazan H, Lerman Y, Shalom V. Correlates and predictors of loneliness in older-adults: a review of quantitative results informed by qualitative insights. Int Psychogeriatr 2016;28(4):557-76. doi: 10.1017/S1041610215001532.

[14] World Health Organisation. Mexico: Study on global ageing and adult health, 2014, Wave 2. URL: http://apps.who.int/healthinfo/systems/surveydata/index.php/catalog/212/datafile/F2/?offset=1000&limit=100.

[15] Filmer D, Pritchett LH. Estimating wealth effects without expenditure data—or tears: an application to educational enrollments in states of India. Demography 2001;38(1):115–32.

[16] Ramlagan S, Peltzer K, Phaswana-Mafuya N. Social capital and health among older adults in South Africa. BMC Geriatr 2013;13:100. doi: 10.1186/1471-2318-13-100.

[17] Bull FC, Maslin TS, Armstrong T. Global physical activity questionnaire (GPAQ): nine country reliability and validity study. J Phys Act Health 2009;6(6):790–804.

[18] US Department of Health and Human Services and US Department of Agriculture. *2015- 2020 dietary guidelines for Americans,* 2015, appendix alcohol. URL: https://health.gov/our-work/food-nutrition/2015-2020-dietary-guidelines/guidelines/appendix-9/.

[19] World Health Organization. Guidelines for controlling and monitoring the tobacco epidemic. Geneva, Switzerland: WHO, 1998.

[20] Vancampfort D, Stubbs B, Koyanagi A. Physical chronic conditions, multimorbidity and sedentary behavior amongst middle-aged and older adults in six low- and middle-income countries. Int J Behav Nutr Phys Act 2017;14(1):147. doi: 10.1186/s12966-017-0602-z.

[21] Rose GA. The diagnosis of ischaemic heart pain and intermittent claudication in field surveys. Bull World Health Organ 1962;27:645–58.

[22] Peltzer K, Hewlett S, Yawson AE, Moynihan P, Preet R, Wu F, et al. Prevalence of loss of all teeth (edentulism) and associated factors in older adults in China, Ghana,

India, Mexico, Russia and South Africa. Int J Environ Res Public Health 2014;11(11):11308–24. https://doi.org/10.3390/ijerph111111308.

[23] Chobanian AV, Bakris GL, Black HR, Cushman WC, Green LA, Izzo Jr JL, et al. The seventh report of the joint national committee on prevention, detection, evaluation, and treatment of high blood pressure: The JNC 7 report. JAMA 2003;289(19):2560–71.

[24] Arokiasamy P, Uttamacharya, Kowal P, Capistrant BD, Gildner TE, Thiele E, et al. Chronic noncommunicable diseases in 6 low- and middle-income countries: findings from wave 1 of the World Health Organization's Study on Global Ageing and Adult Health (SAGE). Am J Epidemiol 2017;185(6):414-28. doi: 10.1093/aje/kww125.

[25] Ustün T, Kostanjsek N, Chatterji S, Rehm J, eds. Measuring health and disability: Manual for WHO Disability Assessment Schedule (WHODAS 2.0). Geneva, Switzerland: WHO, 2010.

[26] World Health Organisation. World report on disability. Malta: WHO, 2011.

[27] Poscia A, Stojanovic J, La Milia DI, Duplaga M, Grysztar M, Moscato U, et al. Interventions targeting loneliness and social isolation among the older people: An update systematic review. Exp Gerontol 2018;102:133-44. doi: 10.1016/j.exger. 2017.11.017.

[28] Kamiya Y, Doyle M, Henretta JC, Timonen V. Early-life circumstances and later-life loneliness in Ireland. Gerontologist 2014;54(5):773–83. https:// doi.org/10.1093/geront/gnt097.

[29] Nyqvist F, Victor CR, Forsman AK, Cattan M. The association between social capital and loneliness in diferent age groups: a populationbased study in Western Finland. BMC Public Health 2016;16:542. https ://doi.org/10.1186/s12889-016-3248-x.

[30] Victor CR, Yang K. The prevalence of loneliness among adults: a case study of the United Kingdom. J Psychol 2012;146(1–2):85–104. https:// doi.org/10.1080/ 00223980.2011.613875.

[31] Jessen MAB, Pallesen AVJ, Kriegbaum M, Kristiansen M. The association between loneliness and health—a survey-basedstudy among middleaged and older adults in Denmark. Aging Ment Health 2018;22(10):1338-43. https://doi. org/10.1080/ 13607863.2017.1348480.

[32] Vancampfort D, Lara E, Smith L, Rosenbaum S, Firth J, Stubbs B, et al. Physical activity and loneliness among adults aged 50 years or older in six low- and middle-income countries. Int J Geriatr Psychiatry 2019;34(12):1855-64. doi: 10.1002/gps.5202.

[33] Richard A, Rohrmann S, Vandeleur CL, Schmid M, Barth J, Eichholzer M. Loneliness is adversely associated with physical and mental health and lifestyle factors: Results from a Swiss national survey. PLoS One 2017;12(7):e0181442. https://doi.org/10.1371/journal.pone.0181442.

[34] Hawkley LC, Thisted RA, Cacioppo JT. Loneliness predicts reduced physical activity: cross-sectional & longitudinal analyses. Health Psychol 2009;28(3):354–63. https://doi.org/10.1037/a0014400.

[35] Stickley A, Koyanagi A, Leinsalu M, Ferlander S, Sabawoon W, McKee M. Loneliness and health in Eastern Europe: fndings from Moscow, Russia. Public Health 2015;129(4):403–10. https://doi.org/10.1016/j. puhe.2014.12.021.

In: Mexico: Health and Aging
Editors: Supa Pengpid et al.
ISBN: 978-1-53617-950-7

Chapter 12

PREVALENCE AND CORRELATES OF EDENTULISM IN A NATIONAL SAMPLE OF OLDER ADULTS IN MEXICO

Supa Pengpid[1,2], DrPH and Karl Peltzer[2,*], PhD
[1]ASEAN Institute for Health Development,
Mahidol University, Salaya, Phutthamonthon,
Nakhon Pathom, Thailand
[2]Department of Research Administration and Development,
University of Limpopo, Turfloop, South Africa

ABSTRACT

This chapter aim to determine the prevalence and correlates of edentulism older Mexicans. The study is based on a national population-based cross-sectional survey of older adults (50 years and older) (SAGE wave 2-2014-15) in Mexico. Edentulism was assessed by self-report. The sample included 3,903 older adults (50 years and older), with a median age of 61

---

* Correspondence: Professor Karl Peltzer, Department of Research Administration and Development, University of Limpopo, Turfloop Campus, Private Bag X1106, Sovenga 0727, South Africa. Email: kfpeltzer@gmail.com.

years. Results indicate that the prevalence of edentulism was 16.6%, 12.4% in men and 19.9% in women. In adjusted logistic regression analysis, older age, female sex, diabetes and depression were positively associated with edentulism. In sex stratified adjusted logistic regression, among men functional disability and among women arthritis were associated with edentulism. Almost two in five older adults in Mexico have edentulism. Several risk factors were identified, which can be targeted in public health interventions.

INTRODUCTION

Edentulism (=having lost all of one's natural teeth) is a significant public health problem globally because of its high prevalence (>10% in individuals 50 years and older) and related disability (1-3). In a multi-country study in middle-income countries, the overall prevalence of edentulism was 11.7%, ranging from 3.0% in Ghana to 21.7% in 2009/2010 in Mexico (2). In an earlier "National Performance Evaluation Survey" in 2002/2003 the prevalence of edentulism in persons 35 years and older in Mexico was 10.2% (and 30.6% in persons older than 65 years) (4). In a community sample of 70 years and older residents (N = 197) in a district of Mexico City, 23.5% had edentulism (5) and in a cross-sectional investigation of 139 persons 60 years and older "living in long-term care facilities or living independently and participating in adult day care services in the city of Pachuca, Mexico," the prevalence of edentulism was 38.9% (6). There is a lack of more recent national data on the prevalence and correlates of edentulism among older adults in Mexico.

As previously reviewed (3) factors associated with edentulism include "increasing age, female gender, no or lower education, lower economic status, rural residence, smoking, having chronic diseases, diabetes, arthritis, asthma, depression, reduced physical function, functional disability, poor self-rated health and lack of social capital." This study aimed to determine the prevalence and correlates of edentulism in older Mexicans who took part in SAGE wave 2 in 2014.

OUR STUDY

The study is based on a national population-based cross-sectional survey of older adults (50 years and older) (SAGE wave 2-2014-15) in Mexico. The dataset is publically available and study procedures and sampling strategy have been described in detail (7). Briefly, a "stratified multistage cluster sampling design" was used to generate a sample that is nationally representative. Strata were defined by locality (metropolitan, urban, rural). The "Basic Geo-Statistical Areas (AGEB) defined by the National Institute of Statistics (INEGI) constituted the primary sampling units (PSUs) and were selected with probability proportional to size"(7). The individual study response rate was 81% (7).

All procedures performed in studies involving human participants were in accordance with the ethical standards of the Research and Ethics Committees of Mexico's National Institute of Public Health and with the 1964 Helsinki declaration and its later amendments or comparable ethical standards. Informed consent was obtained from all individual participants included in the study (7).

Measures

Edentulism was assessed with the affirmative response to the question, "Have you lost all of your natural teeth?" (2).

Sociodemographic variables included educational level, marital status, age, sex, residence status and wealth quartiles were calculated based on a 19-item household asset list (using principal component analysis) (8).

Self-rated health status was classified, based on the question "In general, how would you rate your health today?" into poor (bad or very bad), moderate (moderate) and good (good or very good).

Functional ability was measured by the "12-item WHO Disability Assessment Schedule, version 2 (WHODAS-II)" (9), with scores of 25-100 indicating moderate, severe or extreme functional disability (10) (Cronbach alpha 0.90).

Angina was assessed with the "World Health Organization's Rose angina questionnaire" (11).

Diabetes was assessed by self-reported diagnosis.

Arthritis and *asthma* were assessed with a symptom-based algorithm (12).

Depression was assessed with asking about depression symptoms in the past 12 months using the "World Mental Health Survey version of the Composite International Diagnostic Interview" (13). Additionally, persons who reported to have taken "any medications or other treatment such as attending therapy or counselling sessions for depression during the last 12 months?" were included in the symptom-based depression.

Current and past daily tobacco use was assessed with the questions, "Do you currently use (smoke, sniff or chew) any tobacco products such as cigarettes, cigars, pipes, chewing tobacco or snuff?" and "In the past, did you ever smoke tobacco or use smokeless tobacco daily?"(14).

Social engagement was measured with nine items on the participation in social activities, e.g., "How often in the last 12 months have you attended any public meeting in which there was discussion of local or school affairs?" Responses ranged from 1 = never to 5 = daily (15). Scores from the nine questions were summed and classified into three groups of low, moderate and high social engagement. (Cronbach alpha 0.65)

Data analysis

Considering the clustered study design, data analyses were conducted with STATA software version 15.0 (Stata Corporation, College Station, TX, USA). Unadjusted and adjusted logistic regression identified predictors of edentulism. P values of below 0.05 were accepted as significant and missing values were excluded from the analysis.

Table 1. Sample and edentulism characteristics

Variable	Sample	Edentulism		
		All	Male	Female
	N (%)	%	%	%
All	3903	16.6	12.4	19.9
Age in years				
50-59	985 (45.1)	7.1	4.7	9.1
60-69	1424 (29.1)	17.7	14.0	20.6
70+	1494 (25.8)	31.9	24.5	37.6
Education				
<Primary	1950 (41.9)	22.1	16.2	26.4
Primary	986 (27.0)	15.3	11.5	17.8
Secondary or more	967 (31.1)	10.2	8.7	11.9
Wealth quartile				
Lowest	954 (21.6)	18.4	11.5	24.2
Low	993 (25.8)	17.5	15.0	19.2
High	1004 (26.2)	17.7	13.0	21.7
Highest	950 (26.4)	13.1	10.2	15.5
Residence				
Rural	1055 (21.2)	15.8	12.8	18.9
Urban	2848 (78.8)	16.8	12.2	20.2
Health and social factors				
Subjective health status				
Poor	348 (7.9)	28.7	22.1	32.7
Moderate	1898 (50.0)	17.1	13.3	19.8
Good	1657 (42.1)	13.7	10.0	17.2
Functional disability	643 (15.6)	26.9	27.0	26.9
Angina	253 (6.4)	24.7	24.0	25.1
Diabetes	944 (23.1)	23.8	18.2	27.9
Arthritis	570 (14.8)	23.1	10.9	29.6
Asthma	157 (4.1)	25.9	25.3	26.2
Depression	442 (11.6)	27.0	15.5	30.8
Past daily tobacco use	294 (6.4)	19.5	16.3	28.0
Daily tobacco use	266 (7.5)	17.5	14.0	25.7
Social engagement				
Low	1418 (38.6)	18.4	14.2	21.4
Moderate	1279 (32.2)	15.9	12.3	18.9
High	1206 (29.2)	14.9	10.4	19.0

FINDINGS

The sample included 3,903 older adults (50 years and older), with a median age of 61 years (15 years interquartile range), 55.7% were female and 44.3% male. About one-third of the participants (31.1%) had secondary or more education, 78.8% were residing in urban areas, 42.1% rated their health status as good, 15.6% had a functional disability and 29.2% were highly socially engaged. Almost one in ten of the older adults (7.5%) were current daily tobacco users, 6.4% were past daily tobacco users, 6.4% had angina, 14.8% arthritis, 4.1% asthma, 11.6% depression and 23.1% diabetes. The prevalence of edentulism was 16.6%, 12.4% in men and 19.9% in women (see Table 1).

Associations with edentulism

In adjusted logistic regression analysis, older age, female sex, diabetes and depression were positively associated with edentulism. In sex stratified adjusted logistic regression among men, functional disability (OR: 2.33, CI: 1.14-4.79) and among women, arthritis (OR: 1.75, CI: 1.07-2.85 were associated with edentulism (see Table 2).

Table 2. Associations with edentulism in older Mexicans

Variable	Adjusted Odds Ratios (95% CI)	Adjusted Odds Ratios (95% CI)
Age in years		
50-59	1 (Reference)	1 (Reference)
60-69	2.82 (1.83, 4.36)***	2.47 (1.63, 3.75)***
70+	6.13 (4.02, 9.34)***	5.21 (3.50, 7.75)***
Gender		
Female	1 (Reference)	1 (Reference)
Male	0.57 (0.42, 0.76)***	0.63 (0.46, 0.85)**
Education		
<Primary	1 (Reference)	1 (Reference)
Primary	0.63 (0.44, 0.90)*	0.82 (0.56, 1.19)
Secondary or more	0.40 (0.27, 0.60)***	0.65 (0.40, 1.06)

Variable	Adjusted Odds Ratios (95% CI)	Adjusted Odds Ratios (95% CI)
Wealth quartile		
Lowest	1 (Reference)	1 (Reference)
Low	0.94 (0.68, 1.31)	(0.68, 1.51)
High	0.96 (0.66, 1.38)	1.07 (0.68, 1.69)
Highest	0.67 (0.45, 0.98)*	0.96 (0.59, 1.57)
Residence		
Rural	1 (Reference)	---
Urban	1.07 (0.66, 1.75)	
Health and social factors		
Subjective health status		
Poor	1 (Reference)	1 (Reference)
Moderate	0.51 (0.36, 0.74)***	0.78 (0.48, 1.27)
Good	0.39 (0.26, 0.60)***	0.74 (0.40, 1.36)
Functional disability	2.15 (1.51, 3.05)***	1.09 (0.69, 1.72)
Angina	1.71 (1.10, 2.68)*	1.30 (0.82, 2.05)
Diabetes	1.86 (1.40, 2.47)***	1.70 (1.23, 2.34)***
Arthritis	1.65 (1.13, 2.41)**	1.33 (0.87, 2.05)
Asthma	1.81 (0.84, 3.87)	---
Depression	2.05 (1.41, 2.98)***	1.77 (1.17, 2.69)**
Past daily tobacco use	1.24 (0.77, 2.00)	---
Daily tobacco use	1.07 (0.70, 1.65)	---
Social engagement		
Low	1 (Reference)	---
Moderate	0.84 (0.62, 1.14)	
High	0.78 (0.55, 1.10)	

CI = Confidence Interval; ***P < .001; **P < .01; *P < 0.5.

DISCUSSION

In this nationally representative sample of older adults in Mexico, the prevalence of edentulism was 16.6%, which is lower than in previous studies in Mexico (2,4-6), but higher than in the six multi-country study (2). It is possible that the Mexican "Specific Program of Oral Health Action 2013-2018" by expanding "health coverage to the most vulnerable communities and raise the quality and promotion of dental care" (16) had an impact on improving oral health.

Consistent with previous investigations (2, 4, 17, 18), that increasing age, female sex and in unadjusted analysis lower education and lower wealth status were associated with edentulism. The higher prevalence of edentulism in women than in men may be related to biological reasons and better dental care attendance (19). Further, lower education and lower wealth status may translate to lower oral health knowledge and less access to oral health care (3). Contrary to some previous studies (20, 21), this study did not find a significant association between low social engagement and edentulism. Functional disability was found in some former research associated with edentulism (2, 3), while in this study this was only found among men. Men with a functional disability may less likely access dental care services (22). Some previous research (22-24) found a relationship between poor self-rated health status and edentulism, while this study only found this in unadjusted analysis.

In agreement with former investigations (2, 17, 25-28), this study found an association between diabetes, depression, and among women arthritis, and in unadjusted analysis angina and asthma. "Whether development of these disorders is causal or casual has not been determined." (25) Unlike some previous research (2, 4, 18), this study did not find an association between tobacco use and edentulism.

Study limitations include the cross-sectional design, the assessment of some variables, including edentulism, by self-report, and that certain relevant variables, such as certain dietary behaviours (e.g., sugar and soft drink intake), knowledge on oral health, were not assessed.

Conclusion

Almost two in five older adults in Mexico had edentulism, and several associated factors were identified, such as female sex, older age, diabetes, functional disability, depression and arthritis, that could assist in programmes promoting oral health.

ACKNOWLEDGMENTS

This paper uses data from WHO's Study on Global Ageing and Adult Health (SAGE). SAGE is supported by the US National Institute on Aging through Interagency Agreements OGHA 04034785; YA1323-08-CN-0020; Y1-AG-1005-0) and through research grants R01-AG034479 and R21-AG034263.

REFERENCES

[1] Tyrovolas S, Koyanagi A, Panagiotakos DB, Haro JM, Kassebaum NJ, Chrepa V, et al. Population prevalence of edentulism and its association with depression and self-rated health. Sci Rep 2016;6:37083. https://doi.org/10. 1038/srep37083.

[2] Peltzer K, Hewlett S, Yawson AE, Moynihan P, Preet R, Wu F, et al. Prevalence of loss of all teeth (edentulism) and associated factors in older adults in China, Ghana, India, Mexico, Russia and South Africa. Int J Environ Res Public Health 2014;11(11):11308–24. https://doi.org/10.3390/ijerph111111308.

[3] Pengpid S, Peltzer K.The prevalence of edentulism and their related factors in Indonesia, 2014/15. BMC Oral Health 2018;18(1):118. doi: 10.1186/s12903-018-0582-7.

[4] Medina-Solís CE[1], Pérez-Núñez R, Maupomé G, Casanova-Rosado JF. Edentulism among Mexican adults aged 35 years and older and associated factors. Am J Public Health 2006;96(9):1578-81.

[5] Castrejón-Pérez RC, Borges-Yáñez SA, Gutiérrez-Robledo LM, Avila-Funes JA. Oral health conditions and frailty in Mexican community-dwelling elderly: a cross sectional analysis. BMC Public Health 2012;12:773. doi: 10.1186/1471-2458-12-773.

[6] Islas-Granillo H, Borges-Yañez SA, Navarrete-Hernández JJ, Veras-Hernández MA, Casanova-Rosado JF, Minaya-Sánchez M, et al. Indicators of oral health in older adults with and without the presence of multimorbidity: a cross-sectional study. Clin Interv Aging 2019;14:219-24. doi: 10.2147/CIA.S170470.

[7] World Health Organisation. Mexico: Study on global ageing and adult health, 2014, Wave 2. URL: http://apps.who.int/healthinfo/systems/surveydata/index.php/catalog/212/datafile/F2/?offset=1000&limit=100.

[8] Filmer D, Pritchett LH. Estimating wealth effects without expenditure data—or tears: an application to educational enrollments in states of India. Demography 2001;38(1):115–32.

[9] Ustün T, Kostanjsek N, Chatterji S, Rehm J, eds. Measuring health and disability: manual for WHO Disability Assessment Schedule (WHODAS 2.0). Geneva, Switzerland: WHO, 2010.

[10] World Health Organisation. World report on disability. Malta: WHO, 2011.

[11] Rose GA. The diagnosis of ischaemic heart pain and intermittent claudication in field surveys. Bull World Health Organ 1962;27:645–58.

[12] Arokiasamy P, Uttamacharya, Kowal P, Capistrant BD, Gildner TE, Thiele E, et al. Chronic noncommunicable diseases in 6 low- and middle-income countries: findings from wave 1 of the World Health Organization's Study on Global Ageing and Adult Health (SAGE). Am J Epidemiol 2017;185(6):414-28. doi: 10.1093/aje/kww125.

[13] Kessler RC, Ustün TB. The World Mental Health (WMH) Survey initiative version of the World Health Organization (WHO) composite international diagnostic interview (CIDI). Int J Methods Psychiatr Res 2004;13(2):93–121.

[14] World Health Organization. Guidelines for controlling and monitoring the tobacco epidemic. Geneva, Switzerland: WHO, 1998.

[15] Kowal P, Chatterji S, Naidoo N, Biritwum R, Fan W, Lopez Ridaura R, et al. Data resource profile: the World Health Organization study on global AGEing and adult health (SAGE). Int J Epidemiol 2012;41(6):1639–49.

[16] Cruz G, Picazzo E. Public oral health policies in Mexico. J Oral Res 2017;6(2):32-3. doi:10.17126/joralres.2017.010.

[17] Ren C, McGrath C, Yang Y. Edentulism and associated factors among community-dwelling middle-aged and elderly adults in China. Gerodontology 2017;34(2):195–207. https://doi.org/10.1111/ger.12249.

[18] Islas-Granillo H, Borges-Yañez SA, Lucas-Rincón SE, Medina-Solís CE, Casanova-Rosado AJ, Márquez-Corona ML, et al. Edentulism risk indicators among Mexican elders 60-year-old and older. Arch Gerontol Geriatr 2011;53:258–62.

[19] Haikola B, Oikarinen K, Söderholm AL, Remes-Lyly T, Sipilä K. Prevalence of edentulousness and related factors among elderly Finns. J Oral Rehabil 2008;35:827-35.

[20] Kim EK, Jung YS, Kim KH, Kim KR, Kwon GH, Choi YH, Lee HK. Social capital and oral health: the association of social capital with edentulism and chewingability in the rural elderly. Arch Gerontol Geriatr 2018;74:100–5. https://doi.org/10.1016/j.archger.2017.10.002.

[21] Hanson BS, Liedberg B, Owall B. Social network, social support and dental status in elderly Swedish men. Commun Dent Oral Epidemiol 1994;22:331–7.

[22] Olofsson H, Ulander EL, Gustafson Y, Hörnsten C. Association between socioeconomic and health factors and edentulism in people aged 65 and older: A population-based survey. Scand J Public Health 2017 Aug 03. https://doi.org/10.1177/1403494817717406.

[23] Saman DM, Lemieux A, Arevalo O, Lutfiyya MN. A population-based study of edentulism in the US: does depression and rural residency matter after controlling

for potential confounders? BMC Public Health 2014;14:65. https://doi.org/10.1186/1471-2458-14-65.

[24] Borda MG, Castellanos-Perilla N, Patiño JA, Castelblanco S, Cano CA, Chavarro-Carvajal D, et al. Edentulism and its relationship with self-rated health: secondary analysis of the SABE Ecuador 2009 Study. Acta Odontol Latinoam 2017;30(2):83-9.

[25] Felton DA. Edentulism and comorbid factors. J Prosthodont 2009;18(2):88-96. doi: 10.1111/j.1532-849X.2009.00437.x.

[26] de Pablo P, Dietrich T, McAlindon TE. Association of periodontal disease and tooth loss with rheumatoid arthritis in the US population. J Rheumatol 2008;35(1):70–6.

[27] Medina-Solís CE, Pontigo-Loyola AP, Pérez-Campos E, Hernández-Cruz P, Ávila-Burgos L, Kowolik MJ, et al. Association between edentulism and angina pectoris in Mexican adults aged 35 years and older: a multivariate analysis of a population-based survey. J Periodontol 2014;85(3):406-16. doi: 10.1902/jop.2013.130186.

[28] Gaio EJ, Haas AN, Carrard VC, Oppermann RV, Albandar J, Susin C. Oral health status in elders from South Brazil: a population-based study. Gerodontology 2012;29:214–23.

In: Mexico: Health and Aging
Editors: Supa Pengpid et al.
ISBN: 978-1-53617-950-7

Chapter 13

PREVALENCE AND CORRELATES OF BACK PAIN AMONG A NATIONALLY REPRESENTATIVE POPULATION-BASED SAMPLE OF OLDER ADULTS IN MEXICO

Karl Peltzer[1], PhD and Supa Pengpid[1,2,*], DrPH
[1]Department of Research Administration and Development, University of Limpopo, Turfloop, South Africa and [2]ASEAN Institute for Health Development, Mahidol University, Salaya, Phutthamonthon, Nakhon Pathom, Thailand

ABSTRACT

This chapter aim to determine the prevalence and correlates of back pain in older Mexicans. The study is based on a national population-based cross-sectional survey of older adults (50 years and older) (SAGE wave 2-2014-15) in Mexico. Back pain was assessed with two self-reported

* Correspondence: Professor Supa Pengpid, ASEAN Institute for Health Development, Mahidol University, 25/25 Phutthamonthon Road 4, Salaya, Phutthamonton, Nakhon Pathom 73170, Thailand. Email: supaprom@yahoo.com.

questions. The sample included 3,903 older adults (50 years and older), with a median age of 61 years. Results indicate that the prevalence of past month back pain was 35.6%, 25.7% 1-29 days and 9.9% all 30 days back pain. In adjusted multinomial logistic regression analysis, female sex, lower education, high-risk obesity, depression, perceived stress, moderate and high physical activity and sedentary behaviour were associated with 1-29 days and/or 30 days back pain. In addition, light or moderate alcohol consumption and current tobacco use were negatively associated with 30 days back pain. Almost two in five older adults in Mexico reported past month back pain. Several risk and protective factors were identified, which can be targeted in public health interventions.

INTRODUCTION

Low back pain is the leading worldwide cause of years lost to disability (1) with a global point prevalence of 9.4% and a growing trend in low- and middle-income countries because of ageing (2). In a six-country study among older adults in low- and middle income settings, the prevalence of past month (any day) back pain ranged from 22.0% in China to 55.7% in Russia, and 35.5% in 2009-2010 in Mexico (3). In a community study among indigenous adult Maya-Yucateco communities in Mexico (N = 1,523), 10.0% were diagnosed with low back pain (4). There is a lack of more recent national data on the prevalence and correlates of back pain among older adults in Mexico.

As previously reviewed (3, 5, 6) risk factors for back pain include sociodemographic factors (female sex, lower education, lower wealth, marital status and rural residence), stress, anxiety, depression, heavy physical load, smoking, alcohol consumption, hypertension, physical inactivity and obesity. This study aimed to determine the prevalence and correlates of back pain in older Mexicans who took part in SAGE wave 2 in 2014.

Our study

The study is based on a national population-based cross-sectional survey of older adults (50 years and older) (SAGE wave 2-2014-15) in Mexico. The dataset is publically available and study procedures and sampling strategy have been described in detail (7). Briefly, a “stratified multistage cluster sampling design” was used to generate a sample that is nationally representative. Strata were defined by locality (metropolitan, urban, rural). The “Basic Geo-Statistical Areas (AGEB) defined by the National Institute of Statistics (INEGI) constituted the primary sampling units (PSUs) and were selected with probability proportional to size” (7). The individual study response rate was 81% (7).

All procedures performed in studies involving human participants were in accordance with the ethical standards of the Research and Ethics Committees of Mexico's National Institute of Public Health and with the 1964 Helsinki declaration and its later amendments or comparable ethical standards. Informed consent was obtained from all individual participants included in the study (7).

Measures

Back pain was assessed with two questions, “Have you experienced back pain during the last 30 days?” and “On how many days did you have this back pain during the last 30 days?” Responses were grouped into no pain, 1-29 days pain and all 30 days in the past 30 days.

Sociodemographic variables included educational level, age, sex, marital and residence status and wealth quartiles were calculated based on a 19-item household asset list (using principal component analysis) (8).

High-risk obesity was measured with the waist circumference (“cut-offs of > = 102 centimetres for men and > = 88 centimetres for women”) (9).

Anxiety was measured with the question: "Overall in the past 30 days, how much of a problem did you have with worry or anxiety?" Anxiety was defined as severe or extreme, as opposed to "none, mild or moderate."

Depression was assessed with asking about depression symptoms in the past 12 months using the "World Mental Health Survey version of the Composite International Diagnostic Interview" (10). Additionally, persons who reported to have taken "any medications or other treatment such as attending therapy or counselling sessions for depression during the last 12 months?" were included in the symptom-based depression.

Perceived stress was assessed with two items from the Perceived Stress Scale (11): "How often have you felt that you were unable to control the important things in your life?" and "How often have you found that you could not cope with all the things that you had to do?" Responses ranged from 1 = never to 5 = very often. Summed scores were divided into 2 = low, 3-5 = moderate and 6-10 = high perceived stress (Cronbach alpha 0.87).

Hypertension was measured based on the average of two blood pressure measurements and defined as "systolic blood pressure greater than or equal to 140 mmHg and/or diastolic blood pressure greater than or equal to 90 mmHg19 and/or self-reported treatment of hypertension with antihypertensive medication currently (the last two weeks before interview)" (12).

Physical activity levels (low, moderate or high) were assessed with the "Global Physical Activity Questionnaire (GPAQ)", it gathers data on three domains of physical activity ("activity at work, travel to and from places, recreational activities") and sedentary behaviour (13).

Sedentary behaviour was measured with one question by the GPAQ on the "time usually spent sitting or reclining on a typical day". Seven or more hours a day was classified as sedentary behaviour (14).

High-risk alcohol use was assessed with the question "During the past 7 days, how many drinks of any alcoholic beverage (such as beer, wine, spirits, etc.) did you have each day?" and defined as "the consumption of 4 or more drinks on any day or 8 or more drinks per week for women and 5 or more drinks on any day or 15 or more drinks per week for men" (15).

Current alcohol use was assessed with past month consumption of drinks that "contain alcohol (such as beer, wine, spirits, etc.)" Responses were classified in no alcohol use in the past month or ever, low-risk alcohol use in the past month and high-risk alcohol use in the past week.

Tobacco use was assessed with the questions, "Have you ever smoked tobacco or used smokeless tobacco?" "Do you currently use (smoke, sniff or chew) any tobacco products such as cigarettes, cigars, pipes, chewing tobacco or snuff?" "In the past, did you ever smoke tobacco or use smokeless tobacco daily?" Responses were grouped into never, past and current (daily or not daily) tobacco use (16).

Data analysis

Considering the clustered study design, data analyses were conducted with STATA software version 15.0 (Stata Corporation, College Station, TX, USA). Adjusted multinomial logistic regression was used to calculate predictors of 1-29 days back pain and 30 days back pain (with no back pain as reference category. P values of below 0.05 were accepted as significant and missing values were excluded from the analysis.

FINDINGS

The sample included 3,903 older adults (50 years and older), with a median age of 61 years (15 years interquartile range), 55.7% were female and 44.3% male. About one-third of the participants (31.1%) had secondary or more education, 66.5% were married or cohabiting, 78.8% were residing in urban areas, 46.7% were physically inactive, 6.7% sedentary behaviour, 12.1% were currently using tobacco, and 11.1% engaged in low-risk alcohol use. Almost two thirds of older adults (61.8%) had high-risk obesity, 29.8% had high perceived stress, 4.9% anxiety, 11.6% depression, and 56.9% had hypertension. The prevalence of past month back pain was 35.6%, 25.7% 1-29 days and 9.9% all 30 days (see Table 1).

Table 1. Sample and back pain characteristics among older Mexicans

Variable	Sample	Back pain in past 30 days		
		None	1-29 days	30 days
	N (%)	%	%	%
All	3903	64.4	25.7	9.9
Age in years				
50-59	985 (45.1)	62.9	26.5	10.6
60-69	1424 (29.1)	64.7	27.2	8.0
70-79	1038 (18.8)	67.5	22.4	10.1
80 or more	456 (7.1)	64.3	23.3	12.4
Gender				
Female	2293 (55.7)	59.0	29.8	11.2
Male	1610 (44.3)	71.1	20.7	8.3
Marital status				
Single/separated/divorced/widowed	1525 (33.5)	62.8	25.9	11.2
Married/cohabiting	2378 (66.5)	65.1	25.6	9.2
Education				
<Primary	1950 (41.9)	62.4	27.8	9.8
Primary	986 (27.0)	63.6	28.4	8.0
Secondary or more	967 (31.1)	67.8	20.5	11.7
Wealth quartile				
Lowest	954 (21.6)	65.8	25.2	9.0
Low	993 (25.8)	61.2	28.4	10.4
High	1004 (26.2)	64.0	26.3	9.7
Highest	950 (26.4)	66.6	23.0	10.3
Residence				
Rural	1055 (21.2)	67.1	25.0	7.9
Urban	2848 (78.8)	63.6	25.9	10.4
Waist circumference				
Low risk	1282 (38.2)	72.5	19.6	7.9
High risk	2131 (61.8)	58.3	30.5	11.1
Anxiety	159 (4.9)	42.1	27.9	30.0
Depression	442 (11.6)	37.8	34.4	27.8
Perceived stress				
Low	1530 (38.5)	75.5	18.2	6.2
Moderate	1268 (31.7)	63.0	26.7	10.3
High	1105 (29.8)	51.5	34.3	14.2
Hypertension	2246 (56.9)	64.4	24.5	11.1
Physical activity				
Low	1966 (46.7)	66.8	24.4	8.8
Moderate	1007 (25.4)	61.3	28.2	10.6
High	930 (27.9)	63.1	25.7	11.2
Sedentary behaviour	310 (6.7)	56.9	21.7	21.4
Alcohol use				
Not in past month	3411 (85.6)	63.3	26.1	10.6
Low risk past month	371 (11.1)	71.0	23.8	5.2
High risk past week	121 (3.2)	71.1	21.5	7.3
Tobacco use				
Never	2941 (74.5)	62.0	27.0	11.0
Past	582 (13.5)	68.6	23.7	7.7
Current	380 (12.1)	74.4	20.3	5.3

Associations with back pain categories

Table 2. Associations with back pain categories in older Mexicans (with no back pain as reference category)

Variable	Back pain past 1-29 days	Back pain all past 30 days
	Adjusted Relative Risk Ratios (95% CI)	**Adjusted Relative risk ratios (95% CI)**
Age in years		
50-59	1 (Reference)	1 (Reference)
60-69	0.91 (0.66, 1.26)	0.65 (0.42, 1.01)
70-79	0.71 (0.49, 1.01)	0.82 (0.53, 1.29)
80 or more	1.19 (0.79, 1.80)	1.51 (0.76, 3.00)
Gender		
Female	1 (Reference)	1 (Reference)
Male	0.72 (0.53, 0.98)*	1.08 (0.61, 1.93)
Marital status		
Single/separated/divorced/widowed	1 (Reference)	1 (Reference)
Married/cohabiting	1.14 (0.86, 1.51)	1.10 (0.73, 1.66)
Education		
<Primary	1 (Reference)	1 (Reference)
Primary	0.92 (0.66, 1.28)	0.71 (0.42, 1.18)
Secondary or more	0.64 (0.43, 0.96)*	0.97 (0.56, 1.70)
Wealth quartile		
Lowest	1 (Reference)	1 (Reference)
Low	1.43 (0.98, 2.08)	1.70 (1.05, 2.75)*
High	1.12 (0.72, 1.76)	1.49 (0.81, 2.75)
Highest	1.13 (0.75, 1.71)	1.68 (0.92, 3.04)
Residence		
Rural	1 (Reference)	1 (Reference)
Urban	1.10 (0.77, 1.57)	1.13 (0.69, 1.84)
Waist circumference		
Low risk	1 (Reference)	1 (Reference)
High risk	1.61 (1.15, 2.26)**	1.34 (0.87, 2.08)
Anxiety	1.11 (0.54, 2.26)	2.41 (1.04, 5.57)*
Depression	1.81 (1.13, 2.92)*	4.20 (2.59, 6.82)***
Perceived stress		
Low	1 (Reference)	1 (Reference)
Moderate	1.66 (1.21, 2.27)**	1.90 (1.16, 3.09)**
High	2.47 (1.73, 3.53)***	2.54 (1.45, 4.42)***
Hypertension	0.78 (0.58, 1.06)	1.19 (0.80, 1.79)
Physical activity		
Low	1 (Reference)	1 (Reference)
Moderate	1.22 (0.85, 1.74)	1.65 (1.07, 2.54)*
High	1.38 (0.99, 1.93)	2.03 (1.30, 3.16)**
Sedentary behaviour	0.95 (0.60, 1.57)	1.60 (1.27, 5.36)**
Alcohol use		
Not in past month	1 (Reference)	1 (Reference)
Low risk past month	1.15 (0.75, 1.76)	0.54 (0.30, 0.99)*
High risk past week	1.01 (0.51, 2.00)	0.80 (0.28, 2.28)
Tobacco use		
Never	1 (Reference)	1 (Reference)
Past	0.93 (0.62, 1.39)	0.63 (0.35, 1.11)
Current	0.70 (0.43, 1.16)	0.37 (0.17, 0.81)*

CI = Confidence Interval; ***P<.001; **P<.01; *P<0.5.

In adjusted multinomial logistic regression analysis, female sex, lower education, high-risk obesity, depression, perceived stress, moderate and high physical activity and sedentary behaviour were associated with 1-29 days and/or 30 days back pain. In addition, light or moderate alcohol consumption and current tobacco use were negative associated with 30 days back pain (see Table 2).

DISCUSSION

In this nationally representative sample of older adults in Mexico, the past month any back pain prevalence was 35.6% (9.9% all 30 days), which is higher than in China but similar to 2009-2010 Mexico survey (35.5%) (3). Connelly et al. (17) propose "behaviour and exercise therapy and lifestyle change, in addition to pharmacological interventions, for the treatment and management for back pain."

Consistent with previous research (3, 6, 18), this study found that female sex and lower education was associated with back pain. "Multiple biological and psychosocial mechanisms" may contribute to the sex differences in back pain prevalence (3). Further, older adults with lower education may be more involved in strenuous physical activities than their more education counterpart, thus contributing to more back pain (3). Older adults in this study who engaged in moderate or high physical activity and sedentary behaviour were more likely to have back pain. In a systematic review, "increased sitting time at work reduces the risk of lower back pain while increased physical activity during work and/or leisure increases the risk of lower back pain"(19), while in another review "prolonged sitting increases immediate reporting of lower back pain in adults" (20).

In line with former research (18, 21), this study found an association between perceived stress, anxiety, depression and back pain. In a previous review (22), overweight and obesity were associated with chronic low back pain, while this was confirmed in this study in case of abdominal obesity. In a meta-analysis, Shiri et al. (23) found that "both current and former smokers have a higher prevalence and incidence of low back pain than never smokers," while this study did not find an association with former tobacco users, and a negative association with current tobacco users. In a systematic review, Ferreira et al. (24) showed that "alcohol consumption appears to be associated with complex and chronic lower back pain only and in people with alcohol consumption dependence," while in this study light or moderate alcohol use was protective against chronic back pain. Study limitations include the cross-sectional design, the assessment of some variables by self-report. Some determinants, such as depression or substance use, may also be consequences. Longitudinal studies are needed to determine causality.

CONCLUSION

Almost two in five older adults in Mexico reported past month back pain. Several risk factors, such as female sex, lower education, high risk obesity, depression, perceived stress, moderate and high physical activity and sedentary behaviour were identified, which can be targeted in public health interventions.

ACKNOWLEDGMENT

This paper uses data from WHO's Study on Global Ageing and Adult Health (SAGE). SAGE is supported by the US National Institute on Aging through Interagency Agreements OGHA 04034785; YA1323-08-CN-0020; Y1-AG-1005-0) and through research grants R01-AG034479 and R21-AG034263.

REFERENCES

[1] Buchbinder R, van Tulder M, Öberg B, Costa LM, Woolf A, Schoene M, et al. Low back pain: a call for action. Lancet 2018;391(10137):2384-8. doi: 10.1016/S0140-6736(18)30488-4.

[2] Hoy D, March L, Brooks P, Blyth F, Woolf A, Bain C, et al. The global burden of low back pain: estimates from the Global Burden of Disease 2010 study. Ann Rheum Dis 2014;73(6):968–74.

[3] Stewart Williams J, Ng N, Peltzer K, Yawson A, Biritwum R, Maximova T, et al. Risk factors and disability associated with low back pain in older adults in low- and middle-income countries. Results from the WHO Study on Global AGEing and Adult Health (SAGE). PLoS One 2015;10(6):e0127880. doi: 10.1371/journal.pone.0127880.

[4] Peláez-Ballestas I, Alvarez-Nemegyei J, Loyola-Sánchez A, Escudero ML. Prevalence and factors associated with musculoskeletal disorders and rheumatic diseases in indigenous Maya-Yucateco people: A cross-sectional community-based study. Clin Rheumatol 2016;35(Suppl 1):15-23. doi: 10.1007/s10067-015-3085-9.

[5] Koyanagi A, Stickley A, Garin N, Miret M, Ayuso-Mateos JL, Leonardi M, et al. The association between obesity and back pain in nine countries: A cross-sectional study. BMC Public Health 2015;15:123. doi: 10.1186/s12889-015-1362-9.

[6] Jesus-Moraleida FR, Ferreira PH, Ferreira ML, Silva JP, Maher CG, Enthoven WTM, et al. Back complaints in the elders in Brazil and the Netherlands: a cross-sectional comparison. Age Ageing 2017;46(3):476-81. doi: 10.1093/ageing/afw230.

[7] World Health Organisation. Mexico: Study on global ageing and adult health, 2014, Wave 2. URL: http://apps.who.int/healthinfo/systems/surveydata/index.php/catalog/212/datafile/F2/?offset=1000&limit=100.

[8] Filmer D, Pritchett LH. Estimating wealth effects without expenditure data—or tears: an application to educational enrollments in states of India. Demography 2001;38(1):115–32.

[9] World Health Organization. Waist circumference and waist-hip ratio. Report of a WHO expert consultation, Geneva, 8-11 December 2008. URL: https://www.who.int/nutrition/publications/obesity/WHO_report_waistcircumference_and_waisthip_ratio/en/.

[10] Kessler RC, Ustün TB. The World Mental Health (WMH) Survey initiative version of the World Health Organization (WHO) composite international diagnostic interview (CIDI). Int J Methods Psychiatr Res 2004;13(2):93–121.

[11] Cohen S, Kamarck T, Mermelstein R. A global measure of perceived stress. J Health Soc Behav 1983;24:385–96. doi: 10.2307/2136404

[12] Chobanian AV, Bakris GL, Black HR, Cushman WC, Green LA, Izzo Jr JL, et al. The seventh report of the joint national committee on prevention, detection,

evaluation, and treatment of high blood pressure: The JNC 7 report. JAMA 2003;289(19):2560–71.
[13] Bull FC, Maslin TS, Armstrong T. Global physical activity questionnaire (GPAQ): nine country reliability and validity study. J Phys Act Health 2009;6(6):790–804.
[14] Shih YH, Chang HY, Lu MI, Hurng BS. Time trend of prevalence of self-reported cataract and its association with prolonged sitting in Taiwan from 2001 and 2013. BMC Ophthalmol 2014;14:128. doi: 10.1186/1471-2415-14-128.
[15] US Department of Health and Human Services and US Department of Agriculture. 2015- 2020 dietary guidelines for Americans, 2015, appendix alcohol. URL: https://health.gov/our-work/food-nutrition/2015-2020-dietary-guidelines/guidelines/appendix-9/.
[16] World Health Organization. Guidelines for controlling and monitoring the tobacco epidemic. Geneva, Switzerland: WHO, 1998.
[17] Connelly LB, Woolf A, Brooks P. Cost-effectiveness of interventions for musculoskeletal conditions. In: Jamison DT BJ, Measham AR, eds. Disease control priorities in developing countries, 2nd ed. Washington, DC: World Bank, 2006.
[18] Hoy D, Brooks P, Blyth F, Buchbinder R. The epidemiology of low back pain. Best Pract Res Clin Rheumatol 2010;24(6):769-81. doi: 10.1016/j.berh.2010.10.002.
[19] Øverås CK, Villumsen M, Axén I, Cabrita M, Leboeuf-Yde C, Hartvigsen J, et al. Association between objectively measured physical behaviour and neck- and/or low back pain: A systematic review. Eur J Pain 2020 Feb 24. doi: 10.1002/ejp.1551.
[20] De Carvalho DE, de Luca K, Funabashi M, Breen A, Wong AYL, Johansson MS, et al. Association of exposures to seated postures with immediate increases in back pain: A systematic review of studies with objectively measured sitting time. J Manipulative Physiol Ther 2020 Feb 17.; pii: S0161-4754(19)30432-4. doi: 10.1016/j.jmpt.2019.10.001.
[21] Manek NJ, MacGregor AJ. Epidemiology of back disorders: prevalence, risk factors, and prognosis. Curr Opin Rheumatol 2005;17(2):134-40.
[22] Shiri R, Karppinen J, Leino-Arjas P, Solovieva S, Viikari-Juntura E. The association between obesity and low back pain: A meta-analysis. Am J Epidemiol 2010;171(2):135-54. doi: 10.1093/aje/kwp356.
[23] Shiri R, Karppinen J, Leino-Arjas P, Solovieva S, Viikari-Juntura E. The association between smoking and low back pain: a meta-analysis. Am J Med 2010;123(1):87. doi: 10.1016/j.amjmed.2009.05.028.
[24] Ferreira PH, Pinheiro MB, Machado GC, Ferreira ML. Is alcohol intake associated with low back pain? A systematic review of observational studies. Man Ther 2013;18(3):183-90. doi: 10.1016/j.math.2012.10.007.

In: Mexico: Health and Aging
Editors: Supa Pengpid et al.
ISBN: 978-1-53617-950-7

Chapter 14

PREVALENCE AND CORRELATES OF ARTHRITIS AMONG A NATIONALLY REPRESENTATIVE POPULATION-BASED SAMPLE OF OLDER ADULTS IN MEXICO

Supa Pengpid*[1,2]*, DrPH and Karl Peltzer*[2,*]*, PhD
[1]ASEAN Institute for Health Development, Mahidol University, Salaya, Phutthamonthon, Nakhon Pathom, Thailand
[2]Department of Research Administration and Development, University of Limpopo, Turfloop, South Africa

ABSTRACT

This chapter aims to determine the prevalence and correlates of arthritis in older Mexicans. The study is based on a national population-based cross-sectional survey of older adults (50 years and older) (SAGE wave 2-2014-15) in Mexico. Self-reported diagnosis and a symptom-based

* Correspondence: Professor Karl Peltzer, Department of Research Administration and Development, University of Limpopo, Turfloop Campus, Private Bag X1106, Sovenga 0727, South Africa. Email: kfpeltzer@gmail.com.

algorithm assessed arthritis. The sample included 3,903 older adults (50 years and older), with a median age of 61 years. Results indicate that the prevalence of self-reported arthritis was 9.2%, and the prevalence of symptom-based arthritis was 14.8%, 17.3% among women and 11.6% among men. In adjusted logistic regression analysis, abdominal obesity, depression and perceived stress were associated with arthritis. In addition, in unadjusted analysis, female sex and sedentary behaviour were positively and current tobacco use was negatively associated with arthritis. About one in seven older adults in Mexico reported arthritis (symptom-based). Several risk factors were identified, which can be targeted in public health interventions.

INTRODUCTION

Arthritis contributes significantly to the global burden of disability (1, 2). The global prevalence of rheumatoid arthritis was 0.24% (2), knee osteoarthritis 3.8% and hip osteoarthritis was 0.85% (1). In a six-country study among predominantly older adults in low- and middle-income settings, the prevalence of self-reported arthritis was 19.9% among women and 14.1% among men (3). In South Africa, the prevalence of self-reported arthritis among older adults was 24.7% (4). In a large "community-based study performed in 5 regions in México," the prevalence of osteoarthritis was 10.5%, "rheumatic regional pain syndromes 3.8%, and rheumatoid arthritis 1.6%" (5). In a study among persons 60 years and older in Mexico City, the of self-reported arthritis was 23.8% (6), and in a study of adults from the "indigenous communities of San Antonio Huitepec and San Carlos Yautepec" (N=1,061) in Mexico, 14.7% were diagnosed with osteoarthritis, 4.9% rheumatic regional pain syndrome and 0.3% rheumatoid arthritis (7). There is a lack of national data on the prevalence and correlates of arthritis among older adults in Mexico.

Risk factors for arthritis may include sociodemographic factors, including female sex (8, 9), older age (9, 10), lower education (11), higher wealth status (9), separated, divorced or widowed (11), rural residence (10), obesity (4, 8, 10), physical inactivity (10-12), sedentary behaviour (13), inadequate fruit and vegetable consumption (14), alcohol use (15) and psychological distress (4, 16, 17). This study aimed to determine the prevalence and correlates of arthritis in older Mexicans who took part in SAGE wave 2 in 2014.

OUR STUDY

The study is based on a national population-based cross-sectional survey of older adults (50 years and older) (SAGE wave 2-2014-15) in Mexico. The dataset is publically available and study procedures and sampling strategy have been described in detail (18). Briefly, a "stratified multistage cluster sampling design" was used to generate a sample that is nationally representative. Strata were defined by locality (metropolitan, urban, rural). The "Basic Geo-Statistical Areas (AGEB) defined by the National Institute of Statistics (INEGI) constituted the primary sampling units (PSUs) and were selected with probability proportional to size" (18). The individual study response rate was 81% (18).

All procedures performed in studies involving human participants were in accordance with the ethical standards of the Research and Ethics Committees of Mexico's National Institute of Public Health and with the 1964 Helsinki declaration and its later amendments or comparable ethical standards. Informed consent was obtained from all individual participants included in the study (18).

Measures

Arthritis was assessed by "self-reported healthcare professional diagnosis, and a symptom-based algorithm" (3). In the symptom-based diagnosis category, "persons who reported having been diagnosed and having received treatment in the last 12 months but did not have the condition based on the algorithm-based" were added to the symptom-based diagnosis category (11).

Sociodemographic variables included educational level, age, sex, marital and residence status and wealth quartiles were calculated based on a 19-item household asset list (using principal component analysis) (19).

High-risk obesity was measured with the waist circumference ("cut-offs of > = 102 centimetres for men and > = 88 centimetres for women") (20).

Anxiety was measured with the question: "Overall in the past 30 days, how much of a problem did you have with worry or anxiety?" Anxiety was defined as severe or extreme, as opposed to "none, mild or moderate."

Depression was assessed with asking about depression symptoms in the past 12 months using the "World Mental Health Survey version of the Composite International Diagnostic Interview" (21). Additionally, persons who reported to have taken "any medications or other treatment such as attending therapy or counselling sessions for depression during the last 12 months?" were included in the symptom-based depression.

Perceived stress was assessed with two items from the Perceived Stress Scale (22): "How often have you felt that you were unable to control the important things in your life?" and "How often have you found that you could not cope with all the things that you had to do?" Responses ranged from 1=never to 5=very often. Summed scores were divided into 2=low, 3-5=moderate and 6-10=high perceived stress. (Cronbach alpha 0.87).

Fruit and vegetable consumption was assessed with two questions: "How many servings of fruits do you eat on a typical day?" and "How many servings of vegetables do you eat on a typical day?" Inadequate FV intake was defined as "less than 5 servings of fruits and/or vegetables a day" (23) (Cronbach alpha 0.65).

Physical activity levels (low, moderate or high) were assessed with the "Global Physical Activity Questionnaire (GPAQ)," it gathers data on three domains of physical activity ("activity at work, travel to and from places, recreational activities") and sedentary behaviour (24).

Sedentary behaviour was measured with one question by the GPAQ on the "time usually spent sitting or reclining on a typical day." Seven or more hours a day was classified as sedentary behaviour (25).

High-risk alcohol use was assessed with the question "During the past 7 days, how many drinks of any alcoholic beverage (such as beer, wine, spirits, etc.) did you have each day?" and defined as "the consumption of 4 or more drinks on any day or 8 or more drinks per week for women and 5 or more drinks on any day or 15 or more drinks per week for men" (26). *Current alcohol use* was assessed with past month consumption of drinks that "contain alcohol (such as beer, wine, spirits, etc.)" Responses were classified in no alcohol use in the past month or ever, low-risk alcohol use in the past month and high-risk alcohol use in the past week.

Tobacco use was assessed with the questions, "Have you ever smoked tobacco or used smokeless tobacco?" "Do you currently use (smoke, sniff or chew) any tobacco products such as cigarettes, cigars, pipes, chewing tobacco or snuff?" "In the past, did you ever smoke tobacco or use smokeless tobacco daily?" Responses were grouped into never, past and current (daily or not daily) tobacco use (27).

Data analysis

Considering the clustered study design, data analyses were conducted with STATA software version 15.0 (Stata Corporation, College Station, TX, USA). Unadjusted and adjusted logistic regression was used to calculate predictors of arthritis. P values of below 0.05 were accepted as significant and missing values were excluded from the analysis.

FINDINGS

The sample included 3,903 older adults (50 years and older), with a median age of 61 years (15 years interquartile range), 55.7% were female and 44.3% male. About one-third of the participants (31.1%) had secondary or more education, 66.5% were married or cohabiting, 78.8% were residing in urban areas, 85.0% ate insufficient fruit and vegetables, 46.7% were physically inactive, 6.7% sedentary behaviour, 12.1% were currently using tobacco, and 11.1% engaged in low-risk alcohol use. Almost two thirds of older adults (61.8%) had high-risk obesity, 29.8% had high perceived stress, 4.9% anxiety and 11.6% depression. The prevalence of self-reported arthritis was 9.2%, and the prevalence of symptom-based arthritis was 14.8%, 17.3% among women and 11.6% among men (see Table 1).

Table 1. Sample and arthritis characteristics among older Mexicans

Variable	Sample	Arthritis self-reported	Arthritis symptom based
	N (%)	%	%
All	3903	9.2	14.8
Age in years			
50-59	985 (45.1)	7.4	13.8
60-69	1424 (29.1)	9.7	15.7
70-79	1038 (18.8)	11.1	14.5
80 or more	456 (7.1)	13.7	17.9
Gender			
Female	2293 (55.7)	13.0	17.3
Male	1610 (44.3)	4.4	11.6
Marital status			
Single/separated/divorced/widowed	1525 (33.5)	11.1	16.9
Married/cohabiting	2378 (66.5)	8.2	13.8
Education			
<Primary	1950 (41.9)	10.0	15.6
Primary	986 (27.0)	8.5	14.1
Secondary or more	967 (31.1)	8.7	14.3
Wealth quartile			
Lowest	954 (21.6)	6.3	13.2
Low	993 (25.8)	11.2	14.9
High	1004 (26.2)	9.1	14.2
Highest	950 (26.4)	9.6	16.5
Residence			
Rural	1055 (21.2)	6.8	12.1
Urban	2848 (78.8)	9.8	15.5
Waist circumference			
Low risk	1282 (38.2)	6.9	9.8
High risk	2131 (61.8)	10.4	18.7
Anxiety	159 (4.9)	22.4	20.0
Depression	442 (11.6)	21.0	30.4

Variable	Sample	Arthritis self-reported	Arthritis symptom based
	N (%)	%	%
Perceived stress			
Low	1530 (38.5)	6.8	9.9
Moderate	1268 (31.7)	8.5	15.9
High	1105 (29.8)	13.1	19.9
Inadequate fruit and vegetable intake	3293 (85.0)	9.1	14.1
Physical activity			
Low	1966 (46.7)	11.5	15.8
Moderate	1007 (25.4)	8.0	14.8
High	930 (27.9)	6.5	13.1
Sedentary behaviour	310 (6.7)	16.5	21.2
Alcohol use			
Not in past month	3411 (85.6)	10.0	15.6
Low risk past month	371 (11.1)	4.7	10.1
High risk past week	121 (3.2)	3.6	10.1
Tobacco use			
Never	2941 (74.5)	10.1	15.8
Past	582 (13.5)	8.4	14.8
Current	380 (12.1)	4.1	8.9

Associations with arthritis (symptom-based)

In adjusted logistic regression analysis, abdominal obesity, depression and perceived stress were associated with arthritis. In addition, in unadjusted analysis, female sex and sedentary behaviour were positively and current tobacco use was negatively associated with arthritis (see Table 2).

Table 2. Associations with arthritis (symptom-based) in older Mexicans

Variable	Unadjusted Odds Ratios (95% CI)	Adjusted Odds Ratios (95% CI)
Age in years		
50-59	1 (Reference)	---
60-69	1.16 (0.81, 1.66)	
70-79	1.06 (0.76, 1.49)	
80 or more	1.35 (0.89, 2.05)	

Table 2. (Continued)

Variable	Unadjusted Odds Ratios (95% CI)	Adjusted Odds Ratios (95% CI)
Gender		
Female	1 (Reference)	1 (Reference)
Male	0.63 (0.47, 0.84)**	0.78 (0.55, 1.11)
Marital status		
Single/separated/divorced/widowed	1 (Reference)	---
Married/cohabiting	0.79 (0.56, 1.10)	
Education		
<Primary	1 (Reference)	---
Primary	0.88 (0.60, 1.31)	
Secondary or more	0.91 (0.63, 1.30)	
Wealth quartile		
Lowest	1 (Reference)	---
Low	1.15 (0.76, 1.74)	
High	1.09 (0.69, 1.73)	
Highest	1.30 (0.82, 2.06)	
Residence		
Rural	1 (Reference)	---
Urban	1.33 (0.94, 1.89)	
Abdominal obesity	2.11 (1.57, 2.84)***	1.79 (1.27, 2.51)***
Anxiety	1.48 (0.73, 2.97)	---
Depression	2.98 (2.10, 4.22)***	2.32 (1.59, 3.40)***
Perceived stress		
Low	1 (Reference)	1 (Reference)
Moderate	1.73 (1.23, 2.42)**	1.75 (1.24, 2.45)***
High	2.27 (1.58, 3.26)***	1.88 (1.28, 2.75)***
Inadequate fruit and vegetable intake	0.71 (0.47, 1.09)	---
Physical activity		
Low	1 (Reference)	---
Moderate	0.93 (0.63, 1.35)	
High	0.80 (0.54, 1.17)	
Sedentary behaviour	1.60 (1.03, 2.50)*	1.49 (0.82, 2.71)
Alcohol use		
Not in past month	1 (Reference)	---
Low risk past month	0.61 (0.36, 1.03)	
High risk past week	0.61 (0.31, 1.21)	
Tobacco use		
Never	1 (Reference)	1 (Reference)
Past	0.93 (0.64, 1.34)	1.03 (0.69, 1.55)
Current	0.52 (0.27, 1.00)*	0.58 (0.29, 1.18)

CI=Confidence Interval; ***P<.001; **P<.01; *P<0.5.

DISCUSSION

In this nationally representative sample of older adults in Mexico, the prevalence of self-reported arthritis was 9.2%, and the prevalence of symptom-based arthritis was 14.8%, which is lower than in the six-country study among predominantly older adults in low- and middle income settings (3, 4), and in a study older adults in Mexico City (6), but similar to the large "community-based study in five regions in México" (5), and in a study of adults from the indigenous communities in Mexico (7). In agreement with previous studies (8, 9), this study found female sex in unadjusted analysis increased the odds for arthritis. While some studies (9-11) found an association between older age, lower education, higher wealth status, separated, divorced or widowed civil status and rural residence, this study did not find any of these association.

Consistent with previous research (4, 8, 10), this study found an association between abdominal obesity and arthritis. Obesity may "exhibit a chronic subclinical inflammatory state" increasing the risk for rheumatoid arthritis (28). Several studies showed an association between lifestyle factors (physical inactivity, sedentary behaviour, inadequate fruit and vegetable consumption and alcohol use (10-14), but this study only found in unadjusted analysis an association between sedentary behaviour and arthritis. "Sedentary behaviour may exacerbate already heightened inflammation in rheumatoid arthritis and hold relevance for disease related outcomes" (13). Further, the study found strong associations between perceived stress, depression and arthritis. Previous studies have shown the role of psychological distress in arthritis (4, 16, 17). Prothero et al. (16) showed that "psychological interventions resulted in small to moderate improvements in biopsychosocial outcomes for patients with rheumatoid arthritis in addition to those achieved by standard care." Study limitations include the cross-sectional design, the assessment of some variables by self-report. Some determinants, such as depression or substance use, may also be consequences. Longitudinal studies are needed to determine causality.

Conclusion

About one in seven older adults in Mexico reported arthritis (symptom-based). Several risk factors, such as high risk obesity, depression, perceived stress and in unadjusted analysis, female sex and sedentary behaviour were identified, which can be targeted in public health interventions.

Acknowledgment

This paper uses data from WHO's Study on Global Ageing and Adult Health (SAGE). SAGE is supported by the US National Institute on Aging through Interagency Agreements OGHA 04034785; YA1323-08-CN-0020; Y1-AG-1005-0) and through research grants R01-AG034479 and R21-AG034263.

References

[1] Cross M, Smith E, Hoy D, Nolte S, Ackerman I, Fransen M, et al. The global burden of hip and knee osteoarthritis: estimates from the global burden of disease 2010 study. Ann Rheum Dis 2014;73(7):1323–30. doi:10.1136/annrheumdis-2013-204763.

[2] Cross M, Smith E, Hoy D, Carmona L, Wolfe F, Vos T, et al. The global burden of rheumatoid arthritis: estimates from the global burden of disease 2010 study. Ann Rheum Dis 2014;73(7):1316–22. doi:10.1136/annrheumdis-2013-204627.

[3] Brennan-Olsen SL, Cook S, Leech MT, Bowe SJ, Kowal P, Naidoo N, et al. Prevalence of arthritis according to age, sex and socioeconomic status in six low and middle income countries: analysis of data from the World Health Organization study on global AGEing and adult health (SAGE) Wave 1. BMC Musculoskelet Disord 2017;18(1):271. doi: 10.1186/s12891-017-1624-z.

[4] Peltzer K, Phaswana-Mafuya N. Arthritis and associated factors in older adults in South Africa. Turk J Geriatr 2013;16(4):389-94.

[5] Peláez-Ballestas I, Sanin LH, Moreno-Montoya J, Alvarez-Nemegyei J, Burgos-Vargas R, Garza-Elizondo M, et al. Epidemiology of the rheumatic diseases in

Mexico. A study of 5 regions based on the COPCORD methodology. J Rheumatol Suppl 2011;86:3–8.

[6] Al Snih S, Ray L, Markides KS. Prevalence of self-reported arthritis among elders from Latin America and the Caribbean and among Mexican Americans from the southwestern United States. J Aging Health 2006;18(2):207-23.

[7] Julián-Santiago F, García-García C, García-Olivera I, Goycochea-Robles MV, Pelaez-Ballestas I. Epidemiology of rheumatic diseases in Mixtec and Chontal indigenous communities in Mexico: a cross-sectional community-based study. Clin Rheumatol 2016;35 Suppl 1(Suppl 1):35–42.

[8] Silverwood V, Blagojevic-Bucknall M, Jinks C, Jordan JL, Protheroe J, Jordan KP. Current evidence on risk factors for knee osteoarthritis in older adults: a systematic review and meta-analysis. Osteoarthritis Cartilage 2015;23(4):507–15. doi:10.1016/j.joca.2014.11.019.

[9] Nakua EK, Otupiri E, Dzomeku VM, Owusu-Dabo E, Agyei-Baffour P, Yawson AE, et al. Gender disparities of chronic musculoskeletal disorder burden in the elderly Ghanaian population: study on global ageing and adult health (SAGE WAVE 1). BMC Musculoskelet Disord 2015;16:204. doi: 10.1186/s12891-015-0666-3.

[10] Patel S, Ram F, Patel SK, Kumar K. Association of behavioral risk factors with self-reported and symptom or measured chronic diseases among adult population (18-69 years) in India: evidence from SAGE study. BMC Public Health 2019;19(1):560. doi:10.1186/s12889-019-6953-4.

[11] Arokiasamy P, Uttamacharya, Kowal P, Capistrant BD, Gildner TE, Thiele E, et al. Chronic noncommunicable diseases in 6 low- and middle-income countries: findings from wave 1 of the world health organization's Study on Global Ageing and Adult Health (SAGE). Am J Epidemiol 2017;185(6):414-28. https://doi.org/10.1093/aje/kww125.

[12] Tierney M, Fraser A, Kennedy N. Physical activity in rheumatoid arthritis: a systematic review. J Phys Act Health 2012;9(7):1036–48. doi:10.1123/jpah.9.7.1036.

[13] Fenton SAM, Veldhuijzen van Zanten JJCS, Duda JL, Metsios GS, Kitas GD. Sedentary behaviour in rheumatoid arthritis: definition, measurement and implications for health. Rheumatology. 2018;57(2):213–26. doi:10.1093/rheumatology/kex053.

[14] Pattison DJ, Harrison RA, Symmons DP. The role of diet in susceptibility to rheumatoid arthritis: a systematic review. J Rheumatol 2004;31(7):1310–9.

[15] Scott IC, Tan R, Stahl D, Steer S, Lewis CM, Cope AP. The protective effect of alcohol on developing rheumatoid arthritis: a systematic review and meta-analysis. Rheumatology 2013;52(5):856–67. doi:10.1093/rheumatology/kes376.

[16] Prothero L, Barley E, Galloway J, Georgopoulou S, Sturt J. The evidence base for psychological interventions for rheumatoid arthritis: A systematic review of reviews. Int J Nurs Stud 2018;82:20–9. doi:10.1016/j.ijnurstu.2018.03.008.

[17] Machado GM, Barreto SM, Passos VM, Lima-Costa MF. Health status indicators among community-dwelling elders with arthritis: the Bambuí health and aging study. J Rheumatol. 2006;33(2):342–7.

[18] World Health Organisation. Mexico: Study on global ageing and adult health, 2014, Wave 2. URL: http://apps.who.int/healthinfo/systems/surveydata/index.php/catalog/212/datafile/F2/?offset=1000&limit=100.

[19] Filmer D, Pritchett LH. Estimating wealth effects without expenditure data—or tears: an application to educational enrollments in states of India. Demography 2001;38(1):115–32.

[20] World Health Organization. Waist circumference and waist-hip ratio. Report of a WHO expert consultation, Geneva, 8-11 December 2008. URL: https://www.who.int/nutrition/publications/obesity/WHO_report_waistcircumference_and_waisthip_ratio/en/.

[21] Kessler RC, Ustün TB. The World Mental Health (WMH) Survey initiative version of the World Health Organization (WHO) composite international diagnostic interview (CIDI). Int J Methods Psychiatr Res 2004;13(2):93–121.

[22] Cohen S, Kamarck T, Mermelstein R. A global measure of perceived stress. J Health Soc Behav 1983;24:385–96. doi: 10.2307/2136404.

[23] World Health Organization. Diet, nutrition, and the prevalence of chronic diseases. Geneva, Switzerland: WHO, 2003.

[24] Bull FC, Maslin TS, Armstrong T. Global physical activity questionnaire (GPAQ): nine country reliability and validity study. J Phys Act Health 2009;6(6):790–804.

[25] Shih YH, Chang HY, Lu MI, Hurng BS. Time trend of prevalence of self-reported cataract and its association with prolonged sitting in Taiwan from 2001 and 2013. BMC Ophthalmol 2014;14:128. doi: 10.1186/1471-2415-14-128.

[26] US Department of Health and Human Services and US Department of Agriculture. *2015- 2020 dietary guidelines for Americans,* 2015, appendix alcohol. URL: https://health.gov/our-work/food-nutrition/2015-2020-dietary-guidelines/guidelines/appendix-9/.

[27] World Health Organization. Guidelines for controlling and monitoring the tobacco epidemic. Geneva, Switzerland: WHO, 1998.

[28] George MD, Baker JF. The obesity epidemic and consequences for rheumatoid arthritis care. Curr Rheumatol Rep 2016;18(1):6. doi:10.1007/s11926-015-0550-z.

In: Mexico: Health and Aging
Editors: Supa Pengpid et al.
ISBN: 978-1-53617-950-7

Chapter 15

PREVALENCE AND CORRELATES OF SHORT AND LONG SLEEP AMONG A NATIONALLY REPRESENTATIVE POPULATION-BASED SAMPLE OF OLDER ADULTS IN MEXICO

Karl Peltzer[1], PhD and Supa Pengpid[1,2,*], DrPH
[1]Department of Research Administration and Development,
University of Limpopo, Turfloop, South Africa
[2]ASEAN Institute for Health Development, Mahidol University,
Salaya, Phutthamonthon, Nakhon Pathom, Thailand

ABSTRACT

In this chapter we wanted to determine the prevalence and correlates of short and long sleep duration in older Mexicans. The study is based on a national population-based cross-sectional survey of older adults (50 years and older) (SAGE wave 2-2014-15) in Mexico. Sleep duration was

* Correspondence: Professor Supa Pengpid, ASEAN Institute for Health Development, Mahidol University, 25/25 Phutthamonthon Road 4, Salaya, Phutthamonton, Nakhon Pathom 73170, Thailand. Email: supaprom@yahoo.com.

assessed with two self-reported questions on the previous two nights. The sample included 3,903 older adults (50 years and older), with a median age of 61 years. Results indicate that the prevalence of short sleep (≤6 hrs) and long sleep (≥9 hrs) was 31.5% and 13.6%, respectively. In adjusted multinomial logistic regression analysis, male sex, chronic lung disease and depression were associated with short sleep, and older age, being single, separated, divorced or widowed and lower education were associated with long sleep). In addition, in unadjusted analysis, anxiety and functional disability were associated with short sleep, and female sex, lower wealth, rural residence, physical inactivity and functional disability were associated with long sleep. Almost one in three and almost one in seven older adults in Mexico reported short and long sleep, respectively. Several risk factors were identified, which can be targeted in public health interventions.

INTRODUCTION

Both short sleep (≤6 hours) and long sleep (≥9 hours) have an increased risk of morbidity and mortality (1, 2). The prevalence of short sleep among older adults (50 years and older) was 11.4% in South Africa (3), 20.3% in China and 29.3% in India (4), and the prevalence of long sleep was 14.9% in India, 25.9% in China (4) and 43.5% in South Africa (3). In a cross-sectional community-based study in "persons 40 years and older in Mexico City, Montevideo, Santiago, and Caracas," the prevalence of short sleep was 38.4% and the prevalence of long sleep 10.2% (5). There is a lack of national data on the prevalence and correlates of short and long sleep among older adults in Mexico.

Several risk factors associated with short sleep have been identified, as reviewed in (6, 7), including low socioeconomic status, female sex, older age, inadequate fruit and vegetable intake, physical inactivity, current tobacco use, cardiovascular disease, diabetes, depression, chronic pain, obesity and functional disability. Likewise, risk factors associated with long sleep, as reviewed in (6, 7), include age, higher education, low socioeconomic status, inadequate fruit and vegetable intake, current smoking, physical inactivity, alcohol use, cardiovascular disease, diabetes, depression, chronic pain and functional disability. This study aimed to determine the prevalence and correlates of short and long sleep in older Mexicans who took part in SAGE wave 2 in 2014.

OUR STUDY

The study is based on a national population-based cross-sectional survey of older adults (50 years and older) (SAGE wave 2-2014-15) in Mexico. The dataset is publically available and study procedures and sampling strategy have been described in detail (8). Briefly, a "stratified multistage cluster sampling design" was used to generate a sample that is nationally representative. Strata were defined by locality (metropolitan, urban, rural). The "Basic Geo-Statistical Areas (AGEB) defined by the National Institute of Statistics (INEGI) constituted the primary sampling units (PSUs) and were selected with probability proportional to size" (8). The individual study response rate was 81% (8).

All procedures performed in studies involving human participants were in accordance with the ethical standards of the Research and Ethics Committees of Mexico's National Institute of Public Health and with the 1964 Helsinki declaration and its later amendments or comparable ethical standards. Informed consent was obtained from all individual participants included in the study (8).

Measures

Sleep duration was measured with two "questions about self-reported hours of sleep last night and the night before last: How many hours (and minutes) did you sleep?" "The sleep duration of the two nights was averaged and categorized sleep hours into ≤6, 7-8, and ≥9 hours per day" (9, 10).

Sociodemographic variables included educational level, age, sex, marital and residence status and wealth quartiles were calculated based on a 19-item household asset list (using principal component analysis) (11).

Food insecurity was assessed with two questions: "In the last 12 months, how often did you ever eat less than you felt you should because there wasn't enough food?" and "In the last 12 months, were you ever hungry, but didn't eat because you couldn't afford enough food?" (Cronbach alpha 0.88). Responses were grouped into no or low, moderate and high food insecurity.

Physical activity levels (low, moderate or high) were assessed with the "Global Physical Activity Questionnaire (GPAQ)," it gathers data on three domains of physical activity ("activity at work, travel to and from places, recreational activities") and sedentary behaviour (12).

High-risk alcohol use was assessed with the question "During the past 7 days, how many drinks of any alcoholic beverage (such as beer, wine, spirits, etc.) did you have each day?" and defined as "the consumption of 4 or more drinks on any day or 8 or more drinks per week for women and 5 or more drinks on any day or 15 or more drinks per week for men" (13). *Current alcohol use* was assessed with past month consumption of drinks that "contain alcohol (such as beer, wine, spirits, etc.)" Responses were classified in no alcohol use in the past month or ever, low-risk alcohol use in the past month and high-risk alcohol use in the past week.

Tobacco use was assessed with the questions, "Have you ever smoked tobacco or used smokeless tobacco?" "Do you currently use (smoke, sniff or chew) any tobacco products such as cigarettes, cigars, pipes, chewing tobacco or snuff?" "In the past, did you ever smoke tobacco or use smokeless tobacco daily?" Responses were grouped into never, past and current (daily or not daily) tobacco use (14).

Fruit and vegetable consumption was assessed with two questions: "How many servings of fruits do you eat on a typical day?" and "How many servings of vegetables do you eat on a typical day?" Inadequate FV intake was defined as "less than 5 servings of fruits and/or vegetables a day" (15) (Cronbach alpha 0.65).

Chronic back pain was defined as "having had back pain every day during the last 30 days" (16).

Hypertension was measured based on the average of two blood pressure measurements and defined as "systolic blood pressure greater than or equal to 140 mmHg and/or diastolic blood pressure greater than or equal to 90 mmHg19 and/or self-reported treatment of hypertension with antihypertensive medication currently (the last two weeks before interview)" (17).

Angina was assessed with the "World Health Organization's Rose angina questionnaire" (18).

Diabetes and stroke were assessed by self-reported diagnosis.

Arthritis, asthma and chronic lung disease were assessed with a symptom-based algorithm (19).

Anxiety was measured with the question: "Overall in the past 30 days, how much of a problem did you have with worry or anxiety?" Anxiety was defined as severe or extreme, as opposed to "none, mild or moderate."

Depression was assessed with asking about depression symptoms in the past 12 months using the "World Mental Health Survey version of the Composite International Diagnostic Interview" (20). Additionally, persons who reported to have taken "any medications or other treatment such as attending therapy or counselling sessions for depression during the last 12 months?" were included in the symptom-based depression.

Anthropometry. Weight and height were measured using standard procedures. Body mass index (BMI) was calculated and obesity defined as $\geq$30 kg/m^2 (BMI) (21).

Functional ability was measured by the "12-item WHO Disability Assessment Schedule, version 2 (WHODAS-II)" (22), with scores of 25-100 indicating moderate, severe or extreme functional disability (23) (Cronbach alpha 0.90).

Data analysis

Considering the clustered study design, data analyses were conducted with STATA software version 15.0 (Stata Corporation, College Station, TX, USA). Unadjusted and adjusted multinomial logistic regression was used to calculate predictors of short sleep ($\leq$6 hrs) and long sleep ($\geq$9 hrs), with medium sleep (7-8 hrs) as reference category. P values of below 0.05 were accepted as significant and missing values were excluded from the analysis.

FINDINGS

The sample included 3,903 older adults (50 years and older), with a median age of 61 years (15 years interquartile range), 55.7% were female and 44.3% male. About one-third of the participants (31.1%) had secondary or more education, 66.5% were married or cohabiting, 78.8% were residing in urban areas, 46.7% were physically inactive, 12.1% were currently using tobacco, 11.1% engaged in low-risk alcohol use and 85.0% ate inadequate fruit and vegetables. One in ten older adults (9.9%) had chronic back pain, 56.9% hypertension, 6.4% had angina, 3.1% stroke, 14.8% arthritis, 4.1% asthma, 11.8% chronic lung disease, 23.1% diabetes, 4.9% had anxiety, 11.6% had depression, and 15.6% had a functional disability. The prevalence of short sleep (≤6 hrs) and long sleep (≥9 hrs) was 31.5% and 13.6%, respectively (see Table 1).

Table 1. Sample and sleep duration characteristics among older Mexicans

Variable	Sample	Medium sleepers	Short sleepers	Long sleepers
	N (%)	%	%	%
All	3903	54.9	31.5	13.6
Age in years				
50-59	985 (45.1)	58.3	32.2	9.6
60-69	1424 (29.1)	54.8	33.3	11.8
70-79	1038 (18.8)	49.3	28.4	22.3
80 or more	456 (7.1)	48.0	27.7	24.2
Gender				
Female	2293 (55.7)	55.2	28.8	16.0
Male	1610 (44.3)	54.5	34.9	10.6
Marital status				
Single/separated/divorced/widowed	1525 (33.5)	51.1	30.6	18.3
Married/cohabiting	2378 (66.5)	56.8	32.0	11.3

Variable	Sample	Medium sleepers	Short sleepers	Long sleepers
	N (%)	%	%	%
Education				
<Primary	1950 (41.9)	49.2	31.8	18.9
Primary	986 (27.0)	56.1	31.6	12.3
Secondary or more	967 (31.1)	61.4	30.9	7.7
Wealth quartile				
Lowest	954 (21.6)	53.3	29.0	17.7
Low	993 (25.8)	48.3	35.0	16.8
High	1004 (26.2)	56.8	30.8	12.5
Highest	950 (26.4)	60.7	30.8	8.5
Food insecurity				
Low	3127 (79.6)	55.5	32.3	12.1
Moderate	535 (13.1)	54.5	27.1	18.4
High	241 (7.3)	48.1	30.3	21.5
Residence				
Rural	1055 (21.2)	53.9	28.3	17.8
Urban	2848 (78.8)	55.1	32.3	12.5
Physical activity				
Low	1966 (46.7)	52.3	32.2	15.5
Moderate	1007 (25.4)	54.9	29.6	15.4
High	930 (27.9)	59.0	32.0	9.0
Alcohol use				
Not in past month	3411 (85.6)	54.9	30.9	14.2
Low risk past month	371 (11.1)	55.4	34.4	10.1
High risk past week	121 (3.2)	52.7	36.9	10.4
Tobacco use				
Never	2941 (74.5)	55.1	30.4	14.4
Past	582 (13.5)	51.2	38.8	10.1
Current	380 (12.1)	57.4	29.9	12.7
Inadequate fruit and vegetable intake	3293 (85.0)	53.3	31.1	13.6
Chronic back pain	372 (9.9)	49.7	38.3	12.0
Hypertension	2246 (56.9)	54.4	30.8	14.8
Angina	253 (6.4)	58.8	29.3	11.9
Stroke	127 (3.1)	53.5	34.0	12.5
Arthritis	570 (14.8)	49.1	36.7	14.2
Asthma	253 (6.4)	48.2	41.3	10.5
Chronic lung disease	427 (11.8)	43.0	43.6	13.3
Diabetes	944 (23.1)	55.1	33.2	11.7
Depression	442 (11.6)	42.7	44.2	13.1
Anxiety	159 (4.9)	40.5	47.8	11.7
Body mass index obesity	1132 (35.5)	57.4	30.7	11.9
Functional disability	643 (15.6)	44.5	38.2	17.3

Table 2. Adjusted associations with sleep duration in older Mexicans

Variable	Short sleep	Long sleep
	Adjusted Relative Risk Ratios (95% CI)	**Adjusted Relative Risk Ratios (95% CI)**
Age in years		
50-59	1 (Reference)	1 (Reference)
60-69	1.06 (0.77, 1.48)	1.22 (0.85, 1.77)
70-79	0.90 (0.65, 1.24)	2.06 (1.29, 3.29)**
80 or more	0.91 (0.58, 1.42)	1.92 (1.23, 3.00)**
Gender		
Female	1 (Reference)	1 (Reference)
Male	1.36 (1.05, 1.77)*	0.77 (0.54, 1.09)
Marital status		
Single/separated/divorced/widowed	1 (Reference)	1 (Reference)
Married/cohabiting	0.91 (0.69, 1.19)	0.67 (0.46, 0.96)*
Education		
<Primary	1 (Reference)	1 (Reference)
Primary	0.90 (0.67, 1.21)	0.74 (0.45, 1.20)
Secondary or more	0.78 (0.53, 1.15)	0.50 (0.31, 0.83)**
Wealth quartile		
Lowest	1 (Reference)	1 (Reference)
Low	1.40 (1.02, 1.94)*	1.46 (0.95, 2.25)
High	1.09 (0.75, 1.57)	1.00 (0.63, 1.57)
Highest	1.09 (0.69, 1.73)	0.85 (0.84, 1.73)
Food insecurity		
Low	1 (Reference)	1 (Reference)
Moderate	0.75 (0.52, 1.08)	1.31 (0.84, 2.04)
High	0.91 (0.55, 1.49)	1.75 (0.88, 3.48)
Residence		
Rural	1 (Reference)	1 (Reference)
Urban	1.16 (0.80, 1.69)	0.81 (0.58, 1.13)
Physical activity		
Low	1 (Reference)	1 (Reference)
Moderate	0.92 (0.66, 1.26)	1.09 (0.70, 1.69)
High	0.91 (0.66, 1.27)	0.71 (0.49, 1.04)
Chronic lung disease	1.73 (1.16, 2.58)**	1.01 (0.56, 1.84)
Depression	1.57 (1.08, 2.27)*	0.91 (0.52, 1.60)
Anxiety	1.49 (0.73, 3.04)	1.10 (0.46, 2.59)
Functional disabilitiy	1.31 (0.90, 1.90)	1.21 (0.84, 1.73)

CI = Confidence Interval; ***P < .001; **P < .01; *P < 0.5.

Associations with short and long sleep

In adjusted multinomial logistic regression analysis, male sex, depression and chronic lung disease were associated with short sleep, and older age, being single, separated, divorced or widowed and lower education were associated with long sleep (see Table 2). In addition, in unadjusted analysis, anxiety and functional disability were associated with short sleep, and female sex, lower wealth, rural residence, functional disability and physical inactivity were associated with long sleep (see Table 3).

Table 3. Unadjusted associations with sleep duration in older Mexicans

Variable	Short sleep Unadjusted Relative Risk Ratios (95% CI)	Long sleep Unadjusted Relative Risk Ratios (95% CI)
Age in years		
50-59	1 (Reference)	1 (Reference)
60-69	1.10 (0.81, 1.51)	1.32 (0.89, 1.95)
70-79	1.05 (0.78, 1.40)	2.76 (1.87, 4.06)***
80 or more	1.05 (0.72, 1.52)	3.08 (1.94, 4.86)***
Gender		
Female	1 (Reference)	1 (Reference)
Male	1.23 (0.95, 1.58)	0.67 (0.50, 0.91)*
Marital status		
Single/separated/divorced/widowed	1 (Reference)	1 (Reference)
Married/cohabiting	0.94 (0.74, 1.20)	0.55 (0.41, 0.75)***
Education		
<Primary	1 (Reference)	1 (Reference)
Primary	0.87 (0.66, 1.16)	0.57 (0.37, 0.87)**
Secondary or more	0.78 (0.58, 1.04)	0.33 (0.21, 0.49)***
Wealth quartile		
Lowest	1 (Reference)	1 (Reference)
Low	1.33 (0.96, 1.85)	1.05 (0.70, 1.56)
High	1.00 (0.69, 1.44)	0.66 (0.41, 1.06)
Highest	0.94 (0.66, 1.32)	0.42 (0.28, 0.62)***
Food insecurity		
Low	1 (Reference)	1 (Reference)
Moderate	0.85 (0.58, 1.26)	1.54 (1.01, 2.35)*
High	1.08 (0.66, 1.77)	2.05 (1.09, 3.84)*

Table 3. (Continued)

Variable	Short sleep	Long sleep
	Unadjusted Relative Risk Ratios (95% CI)	**Unadjusted Relative Risk Ratios (95% CI)**
Physical activity		
Low	1 (Reference)	1 (Reference)
Moderate	0.88 (0.65, 1.18)	0.95 (0.62, 1.45)
High	0.88 (0.63, 1.22)	0.51 (0.37, 0.72)***
Alcohol use		
Not in past month	1 (Reference)	1 (Reference)
Low risk past month	1.10 (0.65, 1.86)	0.71 (0.41, 1.22)
High risk past week	1.24 (0.68, 2.29)	0.76 (0.40, 1.47)
Tobacco use		
Never	1 (Reference)	1 (Reference)
Past	1.37 (0.95, 1.97)	0.75 (0.54, 1.03)
Current	0.94 (0.56, 1.58)	0.85 (0.48, 1.48)
Inadequate fruit and vegetable intake	0.92 (0.66, 1.28)	0.92 (0.61, 1.40)
Chronic back pain	1.39 (0.93, 2.08)	0.96 (0.60, 1.56)
Hypertension	0.94 (0.70, 1.26)	1.24 (0.90, 1.72)
Angina	0.86 (0.54, 1.36)	0.80 (0.37, 1.75)
Stroke	1.11 (0.61, 2.03)	0.94 (0.47, 1.87)
Arthritis	1.37 (0.95, 1.97)	1.19 (0.69, 2.07)
Asthma	1.52 (0.89, 2.60)	0.87 (0.41, 1.83)
Chronic lung disease	1.92 (1.34, 2.75)***	1.28 (0.76, 2.16)
Diabetes	1.06 (0.80, 1.42)	0.81 (0.56, 1.19)
Depression	1.96 (1.35, 2.85)***	1.27 (0.75, 2.25)
Anxiety	2.14 (1.17, 3.89)*	1.17 (0.59, 2.31)
Body mass index obesity	0.90 (0.68, 1.18)	0.80 (0.56, 1.12)
Functional disabilitiy	1.60 (1.15, 2.22)**	1.77 (1.25, 2.53)***

CI = Confidence Interval; ***P < .001; **P < .01; *P < 0.5.

DISCUSSION

In this nationally representative sample of older adults in Mexico, the prevalence of short sleep was 31.5%, which is higher than in previous studies in South Africa (11.4%) (3), in China (20.3%) and in India (29.3%) (4), but was lower than in a study in four major Latin-American cities, including Mexico City (38.4%) (5). The prevalence of long sleep in this study was 13.6%, which is similar to India (14.9%) (4) and the study in

Latin-American cities (5), but lower than in China (25.9%) (4) and South Africa (4).

Some research (24-26) shows that older age is associated with short sleep and younger age is associated with long sleep, while this study found that older age was associated with long sleep. In agreement with a study in Korea (24), this study found that being single, separated, divorced or widowed was associated with long sleep. Some research shows mixed results regarding the association between socioeconomic and residence status and short and/or long sleep (6, 24, 27), while in our study higher education and in unadjusted analysis urban residence were protective against long sleep. In a previous national study among adults in Mexico (28), household food insecurity increased the odds for short sleep, while in this investigation food insecurity increased the likelihood of long sleep.

Some previous studies (6, 7, 24-27, 29) found an association between inadequate fruit and vegetable intake, physical inactivity, alcohol and tobacco use with short and/or long sleep, while this study only found an association between low physical activity and long sleep in unadjusted analysis. Consistent with a previous research, this study found that poor mental health, such as depression and in unadjusted analysis anxiety (6, 24, 30), was associated with short sleep. While in a review (30) depression was also found associated with long sleep, we did not find such association. Nevertheless, the direction of the association between depression and short or long sleep may be bidirectional.

Among various physical chronic conditions (chronic back pain, hypertension, angina, stroke, arthritis, asthma, diabetes, obesity and chronic lung disease), which had been found associated with short and/or long sleep (2, 27, 31), this study only found an association between chronic lung disease and short sleep. Chronic lung disease may increase respiratory symptoms impacting on sleep duration (7). Study limitations include the cross-sectional design, the assessment of some variables by self-report and the assessment of sleep duration was restricted to night-time sleep.

Conclusion

Almost one in three and almost one in seven older adults in Mexico reported short and long sleep, respectively. Several risk factors, such as male sex, chronic lung disease and depression for short sleep, and older age, being single, separated, divorced or widowed and lower education for long sleep, and in unadjusted analysis anxiety and functional disability for short sleep, and female sex, lower wealth, rural residence, physical inactivity and functional disability for long sleep were identified, which can be targeted in public health interventions.

Acknowledgments

This paper uses data from WHO's Study on Global Ageing and Adult Health (SAGE). SAGE is supported by the US National Institute on Aging through Interagency Agreements OGHA 04034785; YA1323-08-CN-0020; Y1-AG-1005-0) and through research grants R01-AG034479 and R21-AG034263.

References

[1] Itani O, Jike M, Watanabe N, Kaneita Y. Short sleep duration and health outcomes: a systematic review, meta-analysis, and meta-regression. Sleep Med 2017;32:246–56. doi:10.1016/j.sleep.2016.08.006.

[2] Jike M, Itani O, Watanabe N, Buysse DJ, Kaneita Y. Long sleep duration and health outcomes: A systematic review, meta-analysis and meta-regression. Sleep Med Rev 2018;39:25–36. doi:10.1016/j.smrv.2017.06.011.

[3] Peltzer K. Sociodemographic and health correlates of sleep problems and duration in older adults in South Africa. S Afr J Psych 2012;18(4):150-6. doi:10.7196/SAJP.369.

[4] Selvamani Y, Arokiasamy P, Chaudhary M. Association of sleep problems and sleep duration with self-rated health and grip strength among older adults in India and China: results from the study on global aging and adult health (SAGE). J Public Health 2018;26:697–707. https://doi.org/10.1007/s10389-018-0906-8.

[5] Torre-Bouscoulet L, Garcia Sancho C, Vázquez García JC, Salazar-Peña CM, Lopez Varela MV, de Oca MM et al. Perceptions of short and long sleep duration and comorbid conditions: the PLATINO study. Sleep Med 2013;14(9):850–7. doi:10.1016/j.sleep.2013.04.014.

[6] Peltzer K, Pengpid S. Self-reported sleep duration and its correlates with sociodemographics, health behaviours, poor mental health, and chronic conditions in rural persons 40 years and older in South Africa. Int J Environ Res Public Health 2018;15(7):1357. doi:10.3390/ijerph15071357.

[7] Krueger PM, Friedman EM. Sleep duration in the United States: a cross-sectional population-based study. Am J Epidemiol 2009;169(9):1052–63. doi:10.1093/aje/kwp023.

[8] World Health Organisation. Mexico: Study on global ageing and adult health, 2014, Wave 2. URL: http://apps.who.int/healthinfo/systems/surveydata/index.php/catalog/212/datafile/F2/?offset=1000&limit=100.

[9] Petrov ME, Lichstein KL. Differences in sleep between black and white adults: An update and future directions. Sleep Med 2016;18:74–81.

[10] Peltzer K. Differences in sleep duration among four different population groups of older adults in South Africa. Int J Environ Res Public Health. 2017;14(5):502. doi:10.3390/ijerph14050502.

[11] Filmer D, Pritchett LH. Estimating wealth effects without expenditure data—or tears: an application to educational enrollments in states of India. Demography 2001;38(1):115–32.

[12] Bull FC, Maslin TS, Armstrong T. Global physical activity questionnaire (GPAQ): nine country reliability and validity study. J Phys Act Health 2009;6(6):790–804.

[13] US Department of Health and Human Services and US Department of Agriculture. *2015- 2020 dietary guidelines for Americans,* 2015, appendix alcohol. URL: https://health.gov/our-work/food-nutrition/2015-2020-dietary-guidelines/guidelines/appendix-9/.

[14] World Health Organization. Guidelines for controlling and monitoring the tobacco epidemic. Geneva, Switzerland: WHO, 1998.

[15] World Health Organization. Diet, nutrition, and the prevalence of chronic diseases. Geneva, Switzerland: WHO, 2003.

[16] Vancampfort D, Stubbs B, Koyanagi A. Physical chronic conditions, multimorbidity and sedentary behavior amongst middle-aged and older adults in six low- and middle-income countries. Int J Behav Nutr Phys Act 2017;14(1):147. doi: 10.1186/s12966-017-0602-z.

[17] Chobanian AV, Bakris GL, Black HR, Cushman WC, Green LA, Izzo Jr JL, et al. The seventh report of the joint national committee on prevention, detection, evaluation, and treatment of high blood pressure: the JNC 7 report. JAMA 2003;289(19):2560–71.

[18] Rose GA. The diagnosis of ischaemic heart pain and intermittent claudication in field surveys. Bull World Health Organ 1962;27:645–58.

[19] Arokiasamy P, Uttamacharya, Kowal P, Capistrant BD, Gildner TE, Thiele E, et al. Chronic noncommunicable diseases in 6 low- and middle-income countries: findings from wave 1 of the World Health Organization's Study on Global Ageing and Adult Health (SAGE). Am J Epidemiol 2017;185(6):414-28. doi: 10.1093/aje/kww125.

[20] Kessler RC, Ustün TB. The World Mental Health (WMH) Survey initiative version of the World Health Organization (WHO) composite international diagnostic interview (CIDI). Int J Methods Psychiatr Res 2004;13(2):93–121.

[21] World Health Organization. The international classification of adult underweight, overweight and obesity according to BMI, 2018. URL: http://apps.who.int/bmi/index.jsp?introPage=intro_3.html.

[22] Ustün T, Kostanjsek N, Chatterji S, Rehm J, eds. Measuring health and disability: Manual for WHO Disability Assessment Schedule (WHODAS 2.0). Geneva, Switzerland: WHO, 2010.

[23] World Health Organisation. World report on disability. Malta: WHO, 2011.

[24] Ryu SY, Kim KS, Han MA. Factors associated with sleep duration in Korean adults: results of a 2008 community health survey in Gwangju metropolitan city, Korea. J Korean Med Sci 2011;26(9):1124–31. doi:10.3346/jkms.2011.26.9.1124.

[25] Wang S, Li B, Wu Y, Ungvari GS, Ng CH, Fu Y, et al. Relationship of sleep duration with sociodemographic characteristics, lifestyle, mental health, and chronic diseases in a large Chinese adult population. J Clin Sleep Med 2017;13(3):377-84. doi: 10.5664/jcsm.6484.

[26] Park S, Cho MJ, Chang SM, Bae JN, Jeon HJ, Cho SJ, et al. Relationships of sleep duration with sociodemographic and health-related factors, psychiatric disorders and sleep disturbances in a community sample of Korean adults. J Sleep Res 2010;19(4):567-77. doi: 10.1111/j.1365-2869.2010.00841.x.

[27] Wang S, Wu Y, Ungvari GS, Ng CH, Forester BP, Gatchel JR, et al. Sleep duration and its association with demographics, lifestyle factors, poor mental health and chronic diseases in older Chinese adults. Psychiatry Res 2017;257:212-8. doi: 10.1016/j.psychres.2017.07.036.

[28] Jordan ML, Perez-Escamilla R, Desai MM, Shamah-Levy T. Household food insecurity and sleep patterns among Mexican Adults: Results from ENSANUT-2012. J Immigr Minor Health 2016;18(5):1093–103. doi:10.1007/s10903-015-0246-5.

[29] Stranges S, Dorn JM, Shipley MJ, Kandala NB, Trevisan M, Miller MA, et al. Correlates of short and long sleep duration: a cross-cultural comparison between the United Kingdom and the United States: the Whitehall II Study and the Western New York Health Study. Am J Epidemiol 2008;168(12):1353-64. doi: 10.1093/aje/kwn337.

[30] Zhai L, Zhang H, Zhang D. Sleep duration and depression among adults: a meta-analysis of prospective studies. Depress Anxiety 2015;32(9):664–70. doi:10.1002/da.22386.

[31] Anujuo K, Stronks K, Snijder MB, Jean-Louis G, Rutters F, van den Born BJ, et al. Relationship between short sleep duration and cardiovascular risk factors in a multi-ethnic cohort - the helius study. Sleep Med 2015;16(12):1482-8. doi: 10.1016/j.sleep.2015.08.014.

In: Mexico: Health and Aging
Editors: Supa Pengpid et al.
ISBN: 978-1-53617-950-7

Chapter 16

PREVALENCE, SOCIAL AND HEALTH CORRELATES OF SLEEP PROBLEMS AMONG A NATIONALLY REPRESENTATIVE POPULATION-BASED SAMPLE OF OLDER ADULTS IN MEXICO

Supa Pengpid[1,2], DrPH and Karl Peltzer[2,*], PhD
[1]ASEAN Institute for Health Development, Mahidol University, Salaya, Phutthamonthon, Nakhon Pathom, Thailand and [2]Department of Research Administration and Development, University of Limpopo, Turfloop, South Africa

ABSTRACT

This chapter aim to determine the prevalence and correlates of sleep problems in older Mexicans. The study is based on a national population-

---

* Correspondence: Professor Karl Peltzer, Department of Research Administration and Development, University of Limpopo, Turfloop Campus, Private Bag X1106, Sovenga 0727, South Africa. Email: kfpeltzer@gmail.com.

based cross-sectional survey of older adults (50 years and older) (SAGE wave 2-2014-15) in Mexico. Sleep problems was assessed with one self-reported question. The sample included 3,903 older adults (50 years and older), with a median age of 61 years. Results indicate that the prevalence of severe/extreme sleep problems was 6.4%, 4.6% among men and 7.9% among women. In adjusted logistic regression analysis, being 80 years and older, urban residence, perceived stress, anxiety, depression and functional disability were associated with sleep problems. In addition, in unadjusted analysis, female sex, being single, separated, divorced or widowed, low trust and multimorbidity were associated sleep problems. More than one in 20 older adults in Mexico reported severe or extreme sleep problems. Several risk and protective factors were identified, which can be targeted in public health interventions.

INTRODUCTION

Sleep disorders affect large populations and have significant public health impacts (1). As people age, the increase in the incidence of chronic diseases, stressful and emotional life events, and the consumption of medications have a substantial impact on sleep quality (2, 3). Approximately 5% of older adults meet criteria for clinically significant insomnia disorders and 20% for sleep apnea syndromes (4). In a cross-sectional survey among older adults (65 years and older) in catchment areas of Mexico in 2003-2006, the prevalence of sleep complaints (based on the question "Have you had trouble sleeping recently?") was 28.7% (2). In a large 10 country study among older adults (50 years and older), the prevalence of "severe/extreme sleep problems" was 9.2% (5), 9.1% in South Africa (6), and in 2009-2010 in Mexico 5.8% (5). In an older investigation (2004) among adults in Mexico City, the prevalence of having moderate or severe sleep problems was 25% (7). There is a lack of more recent national data on the prevalence and correlates of sleep problems among older adults in Mexico.

Several risk factors associated with sleep problems among (mostly) older adults have been identified (reviewed as in 6, 8, 9), including female sex, lower socioeconomic status, widowhood, urban residence, low social support, perceived stress, depression, anxiety, physical illness, multimorbidity, functional disability, physical inactivity, smoking, alcohol use and poor dietary behaviour. This study aimed to determine the prevalence and correlates of sleep problems in older Mexicans who took part in SAGE wave 2 in 2014.

OUR STUDY

The study is based on a national population-based cross-sectional survey of older adults (50 years and older) (SAGE wave 2-2014-15) in Mexico. The dataset is publically available and study procedures and sampling strategy have been described in detail (10). Briefly, a "stratified multistage cluster sampling design" was used to generate a sample that is nationally representative. Strata were defined by locality (metropolitan, urban, rural). The "Basic Geo-Statistical Areas (AGEB) defined by the National Institute of Statistics (INEGI) constituted the primary sampling units (PSUs) and were selected with probability proportional to size" (10). The individual study response rate was 81% (10).

All procedures performed in studies involving human participants were in accordance with the ethical standards of the Research and Ethics Committees of Mexico's National Institute of Public Health and with the 1964 Helsinki declaration and its later amendments or comparable ethical standards. Informed consent was obtained from all individual participants included in the study (10).

Measures

Sleep problems was measured with one item, "Overall in the last 30 days, how much of a problem did you have with sleeping, such as falling asleep, waking up frequently during the night or waking up too early in the morning?" Sleep problems were defined as severe or extreme=1 and none or mild or moderate=0 (5).

Sociodemographic variables included educational level, age, sex, marital and residence status and wealth quartiles were calculated based on a 19-item household asset list (using principal component analysis) (11).

Social engagement was measured with nine items on the participation in social activities, e.g., "How often in the last 12 months have you attended any public meeting in which there was discussion of local or school affairs?" Responses ranged from 1=never to 5=daily. Scores from the nine questions were summed and classified into three groups of low, moderate and high social engagement (Cronbach alpha 0.65).

Trust was measured with five questions, e.g., "Generally speaking, would you say that most people can be trusted or that you can't be too careful in dealing with people?" Scores from the five questions were summed and grouped into low, median and high trust (12) (Cronbach alpha 0.65).

Unsafe environment was assessed with two items, e.g., "In general, how safe from crime and violence do you feel when you are alone at home?" Scores from the two questions were summed and classified into three groups of low, moderate and high unsafe environment (12) (Cronbach alpha 0.66).

Childhood health status was measured with the question "In general, how would you rate your health when you were a child, before the age of 10?" Poor childhood health status was defined as moderate, bad or very bad and good childhood health status as good or very good.

Perceived stress was assessed with two items from the Perceived Stress Scale (13): "How often have you felt that you were unable to control the important things in your life?" and "How often have you found that you could not cope with all the things that you had to do?" Responses ranged from 1=never to 5=very often. Summed scores were divided into 2=low, 3-5=moderate and 6-10=high perceived stress (Cronbach alpha 0.87).

Anxiety was measured with the question: "Overall in the past 30 days, how much of a problem did you have with worry or anxiety?" Anxiety was defined as severe or extreme, as opposed to "none, mild or moderate."

Depression was assessed with asking about depression symptoms in the past 12 months using the "World Mental Health Survey version of the Composite International Diagnostic Interview" (14). Additionally, persons who reported to have taken "any medications or other treatment such as attending therapy or counselling sessions for depression during the last 12 months?" were included in the symptom-based depression.

Multimorbidity was defined as "two or more chronic physical health conditions (angina, arthritis, asthma, chronic back pain, chronic lung disease, diabetes, edentulism, hearing problems, hypertension, stroke, visual impairment)" (15). *Angina* was assessed with the "World Health Organization's Rose angina questionnaire" (16). *Chronic back pain* was defined as "having had back pain every day during the last 30 days." (15). *Edentulism* was assessed with the affirmative response to the question, "Have you lost all of your natural teeth?" (17). *Diabetes and stroke* were assessed by self-reported diagnosis. *Hearing problems* was accepted if "the interviewer observed this condition during the survey."(15) *Visual impairment* was defined as "having severe or extreme difficulty in seeing and recognizing a person that the participant knows across the road." *Hypertension* was measured based on the average of two blood pressure measurements and defined as "systolic blood pressure greater than or equal to 140 mmHg and/or diastolic blood pressure greater than or equal to 90 mmHg19 and/or self-reported treatment of hypertension with antihypertensive medication currently (the last two weeks before interview)" (18). *Arthritis, asthma and chronic lung disease* were assessed with a symptom-based algorithm (19).

Functional ability was measured by the "12-item WHO Disability Assessment Schedule, version 2 (WHODAS-II)" (20), with scores of 25-100 indicating moderate, severe or extreme functional disability (21) (Cronbach alpha 0.90)

Fruit and vegetable consumption was assessed with two questions: "How many servings of fruits do you eat on a typical day?" and "How many servings of vegetables do you eat on a typical day?" Inadequate FV intake was defined as "less than 5 servings of fruits and/or vegetables a day" (22) (Cronbach alpha 0.65).

Physical activity levels (low, moderate or high) were assessed with the "Global Physical Activity Questionnaire (GPAQ)", it gathers data on three domains of physical activity ("activity at work, travel to and from places, recreational activities") (23).

High-risk alcohol use was assessed with the question "During the past 7 days, how many drinks of any alcoholic beverage (such as beer, wine, spirits, etc.) did you have each day?" and defined as "the consumption of 4 or more drinks on any day or 8 or more drinks per week for women and 5 or more drinks on any day or 15 or more drinks per week for men" (24). *Current alcohol use* was assessed with past month consumption of drinks that "contain alcohol (such as beer, wine, spirits, etc.)" Responses were classified in no alcohol use in the past month or ever, low-risk alcohol use in the past month and high-risk alcohol use in the past week.

Tobacco use was assessed with the questions, "Have you ever smoked tobacco or used smokeless tobacco?" "Do you currently use (smoke, sniff or chew) any tobacco products such as cigarettes, cigars, pipes, chewing tobacco or snuff?" "In the past, did you ever smoke tobacco or use smokeless tobacco daily?" Responses were grouped into never, past and current (daily or not daily) tobacco use (25).

Data analysis

Considering the clustered study design, data analyses were conducted with STATA software version 15.0 (Stata Corporation, College Station, TX, USA). Unadjusted and adjusted logistic regression was used to calculate predictors of sleep problems. P values of below 0.05 were accepted as significant and missing values were excluded from the analysis.

FINDINGS

The sample included 3,903 older adults (50 years and older), with a median age of 61 years (15 years interquartile range), 55.7% were female and

44.3% male. About one-third of the participants (31.1%) had secondary or more education, 66.5% were married or cohabiting, 78.8% were residing in urban areas, 46.7% were physically inactive, 29.2% had high social engagement, 29.6% high trust, 40.9% a highly unsafe environment, 29.8% had high perceived stress, and 6.8% had a poor childhood health status. Almost half of the older adults (45.9%) had two or more physical chronic conditions, 85.0% ate inadequate fruit and vegetables, 15.6% had a functional disability, 12.1% were currently using tobacco, 11.1% engaged in low-risk alcohol use, 4.9% had anxiety and 11.6% had depression. The prevalence of severe/extreme sleep problems was 6.4%, 4.6% among men and 7.9% among women (see Table 1).

Table 1. Sample and sleep problem characteristics among older Mexicans

Variable	Sample	Severe/extreme sleep problem
	N (%)	N (%)
All	3903	223 (6.4)
Age in years		
50-59	985 (45.1)	49 (5.0)
60-69	1424 (29.1)	84 (6.6)
70-79	1038 (18.8)	56 (6.6)
80 or more	456 (7.1)	34 (14.7)
Gender		
Female	2293 (55.7)	165 (7.9)
Male	1610 (44.3)	58 (4.6)
Marital status		
Single/separated/divorced/widowed	1525 (33.5)	109 (8.9)
Married/cohabiting	2378 (66.5)	114 (5.2)
Education		
<Primary	1950 (41.9)	114 (6.7)
Primary	986 (27.0)	54 (6.5)
Secondary or more	967 (31.1)	55 (5.9)
Wealth quartile		
Lowest	954 (21.6)	46 (5.4)
Low	993 (25.8)	61 (7.2)
High	1004 (26.2)	52 (6.1)
Highest	950 (26.4)	64 (6.9)
Residence		
Rural	1055 (21.2)	34 (2.4)
Urban	2848 (78.8)	189 (7.5)

Table 1. (Continued)

Variable	Sample	Severe/extreme sleep problem
	N (%)	N (%)
All	3903	223 (6.4)
Social engagement		
Low	1418 (38.6)	116 (8.7)
Moderate	1279 (32.2)	59 (4.4)
High	1206 (29.2)	48 (5.7)
Trust		
Low	1361 (37.0)	104 (8.8)
Medium	1320 (33.4)	66 (6.2)
High	1222 (29.6)	53 (3.8)
Unsafe environment		
Low	1248 (30.0)	51 (4.8)
Moderate	1227 (29.2)	49 (5.9)
High	1428 (40.9)	123 (8.1)
Childhood health status		
Good	3650 (93.2)	197 (6.1)
Poor	253 (6.8)	26 (11.0)
Perceived stress		
Low	1530 (38.5)	39 (2.1)
Medium	1268 (31.7)	71 (6.6)
High	1105 (29.8)	113 (11.8)
Anxiety	159 (4.9)	52 (38.5)
Depression	442 (11.6)	79 (20.3)
Multimorbidity	1840 (45.9)	154 (9.9)
Functional disability	643 (15.6)	94 (17.2)
Inadequate fruit and vegetable intake	3293 (85.0)	187 (6.1)
Physical activity		
Low	1966 (46.7)	136 (7.8)
Moderate	1007 (25.4)	38 (4.9)
High	930 (27.9)	49 (5.5)
Alcohol use		
Not in past month	3411 (85.6)	196 (6.6)
Low risk past month	371 (11.1)	18 (4.4)
High risk past week	121 (3.2)	9 (7.8)
Tobacco use		
Never	2941 (74.5)	169 (6.5)
Past	582 (13.5)	34 (6.9)
Current	380 (12.1)	20 (5.5)

Associations with sleep problems

In adjusted logistic regression analysis, being 80 years and older, urban residence, perceived stress, anxiety, depression and functional disability were associated with sleep problems. In addition, in unadjusted analysis, female sex, being single, separated, divorced or widowed, low trust and multimorbidity were associated sleep problems (see Table 2).

Table 2. Associations with severe/extreme sleep problems in older Mexicans

Variable	Unadjusted Odds Ratios (95% CI)	Adjusted Odds Ratios (95% CI)
Age in years		
50-59	1 (Reference)	1 (Reference)
60-69	1.36 (0.78, 2.37)	1.05 (0.56, 1.99)
70-79	1.36 (0.74, 2.51)	1.13 (0.55, 2.31)
80 or more	2.42 (1.15, 5.09)*	2.48 (1.03, 6.00)*
Gender		
Female	1 (Reference)	1 (Reference)
Male	0.56 (0.34, 0.92)*	0.83 (0.45, 1.52)
Marital status		
Single/separated/divorced/widowed	1 (Reference)	1 (Reference)
Married/cohabiting	0.56 (0.35, 0.89)*	0.79 (0.48, 1.26)
Education		
<Primary	1 (Reference)	---
Primary	0.97 (0.57, 1.64)	
Secondary or more	0.87 (0.49, 1.56)	
Wealth quartile		
Lowest	1 (Reference)	---
Low	1.37 (0.74, 2.56)	
High	1.14 (0.56, 2.34)	
Highest	1.30 (0.66, 2.58)	
Residence		
Rural	1 (Reference)	1 (Reference)
Urban	3.24 (1.65, 6.33)***	2.49 (1.30, 4.77)**
Social engagement		
Low	1 (Reference)	1 (Reference)
Moderate	0.48 (0.30, 0.78)**	0.78 (0.46, 1.30)
High	0.63 (0.34, 1.18)	1.15 (0.53, 2.47)

Table 2. (Continued)

Variable	Unadjusted Odds Ratios (95% CI)	Adjusted Odds Ratios (95% CI)
Trust		
Low	1 (Reference)	1 (Reference)
Medium	0.68 (0.38, 1.22)	0.76 (0.43, 1.25)
High	0.40 (0.25, 0.65)***	0.64 (0.35, 1.18)
Unsafe environment		
Low	1 (Reference)	---
Moderate	1.24 (0.60, 2.56)	
High	1.75 (0.94, 3.25)	
Childhood health status		
Good	1 (Reference)	---
Poor	1.89 (0.87, 4.13)	
Perceived stress		
Low	1 (Reference)	1 (Reference)
Medium	3.32 (1.74, 6.33)***	2.79 (1.41, 5.51)**
High	6.24 (3.75, 10.39)***	3.37 (1.83, 6.22)***
Anxiety	12.40 (7.33, 20.95)***	5.31 (3.05, 9.26)***
Depression	5.25 (3.22, 8.57)***	2.12 (1.27, 3.55)**
Multimorbidity	2.69 (1.71, 4.22)***	1.33 (0.83, 2.13)
Functional disability	4.49 (2.99, 6.73)***	1.80 (1.09, 2.98)*
Inadequate fruit and vegetable intake	0.69 (0.41, 1.17)	---
Physical activity		
Low	1 (Reference)	---
Moderate	0.61 (0.32, 1.14)	
High	0.69, 0.39, 1.21)	
Alcohol use		
Not in past month	1 (Reference)	---
Low risk past month	0.65 (0.35, 1.21)	
High risk past week	1.19 (0.54, 2.59)	
Tobacco use		
Never	1 (Reference)	---
Past	1.06 (0.55, 2.02)	
Current	0.83 (0.37, 1.87)	

CI = Confidence Interval; ***P <. 001; **P < .01; *P < 0.5.

DISCUSSION

In this nationally representative sample of older adults in Mexico, the prevalence of severe or extreme sleep problems was 6.4%, which is higher than in 2009-2010 in Mexico survey among older adults (5.8%) (5), and is lower than the 10 country study among older adults (9.2%) (5), in South Africa (9.1%) (6), and similar to a study among adults in Mexico City with moderate or severe sleep problems of 25% (7), while in this study using the same definition it was 22.7% (analysis not shown).

Some studies (2, 26, 27) found that sleep problems increase with age, which was confirmed in this study with the 80 years and older age group having a prevalence of 14.7% sleep problems compared with 5.0% in the 50-59 year-olds. The increase of chronic conditions with age may contribute to higher sleep problems (28). Most studies (2, 8, 29) find that the prevalence of sleep problems is higher in women than in men, while this was also found in unadjusted analysis in this study. Compared to rural older adults, urban residence had a higher likelihood of having sleep problems in this study. Similar results were found in a previous multi-country study among older adults (2). This may be related to higher stress levels in urban compared to rural areas. In this study urban dwellers had significantly higher perceived stress ($P < 0.25$) than rural dwellers (analysis not shown).

Consistent with previous research results (5, 6, 8, 26), this study showed that perceived stress, depression and anxiety were highly significantly associated with sleep problems. It is possible that "the exposure to different stressors may relate to basic psychological difficulties that affect the sleep pattern negatively" (28). Unlike in a previous study (30), this study did not find an association between adverse childhood (poor childhood health status) and sleep problems. Previous research (2, 5, 6, 8, 9, 30) showed that multimorbidity and functional disability increased the odds for sleep problems, while this study found similar results in unadjusted analysis.

Unlike previous research (2, 8, 27, 30-32), this study did not find any significant association between physical inactivity, tobacco use, alcohol use, poor diet, such as inadequate fruit and vegetable consumption, and sleep problems. This study found in unadjusted analysis that being married or cohabiting, moderate social engagement and high trust were protective against sleep problems. Similar results were found in studies in China (33) and South Africa (6), and shows the importance of social capital in preventing sleep problems. Study limitations include the cross-sectional design, the assessment of some variables by self-report and sleep problems was only assessed with one item. Some relevant variables, such as the consumption of medications, were not assessed, and should be included in futures studies.

CONCLUSION

More than one in 20 older adults in Mexico reported severe or extreme sleep problems. Several risk factors for sleep problems, such as being 80 years and older, urban residence, perceived stress, anxiety depression and functional disability, and in unadjusted analysis, female sex, being single, separated, divorced or widowed, low trust and multimorbidity were identified, which can be targeted in public health interventions.

ACKNOWLEDGMENT

This paper uses data from WHO's Study on Global Ageing and Adult Health (SAGE). SAGE is supported by the US National Institute on Aging through Interagency Agreements OGHA 04034785; YA1323-08-CN-0020; Y1-AG-1005-0) and through research grants R01-AG034479 and R21-AG034263.

REFERENCES

[1] Morin CM, Benca R. Chronic insomnia. Lancet 2012;379(9821):1129-41. doi: 10.1016/S0140-6736(11)60750-2.

[2] Mazzotti DR, Guindalini C, Sosa AL, Ferri CP, Tufik S. Prevalence and correlates for sleep complaints in older adults in low and middle income countries: a 10/66

Dementia Research Group study. Sleep Med 2012;13(6):697–702. doi:10.1016/j.sleep.2012.02.009.

[3] BaHammam A, Pandi-Perumal SR. Interfacing sleep and aging. Front Neurol 2010;1:132. doi:10.3389/fneur.2010.000132.

[4] Gooneratne NS, Vitiello MV. Sleep in older adults: normative changes, sleep disorders, and treatment options. Clin Geriatr Med 2014;30(3):591–627. doi:10.1016/j.cger.2014.04.007.

[5] Koyanagi A, Garin N, Olaya B, Ayuso-Mateos JL, Chatterji S, Leonardi M, et al. Chronic conditions and sleep problems among adults aged 50 years or over in nine countries: a multi-country study. PLoS One 2014;9(12):e114742. doi:10.1371/journal.pone.0114742.

[6] Peltzer K, Pengpid S. Prevalence, and social and health correlates of insomnia among persons 15 years and older in South Africa. South Afr J Psychol 2019;49(4):467-78.

[7] Blanco M, Kriber N, Cardinali DP. A survey of sleeping difficulties in an urban Latin American population. Rev Neurol 2004;39:115–9.

[8] Smagula SF, Stone KL, Fabio A, Cauley JA. Risk factors for sleep disturbances in older adults: Evidence from prospective studies. Sleep Med Rev 2016;25:21–30. doi:10.1016/j.smrv.2015.01.003.

[9] Peltzer K. Sociodemographic and health correlates of sleep problems and duration in older adults in South Africa. S Afr J Psych 2012;18(4):150-6. doi:10.7196/SAJP.369.

[10] World Health Organisation. Mexico: Study on global ageing and adult health, 2014, Wave 2. URL: http://apps.who.int/healthinfo/systems/surveydata/index.php/catalog/212/datafile/F2/?offset=1000&limit=100.

[11] Filmer D, Pritchett LH. Estimating wealth effects without expenditure data—or tears: an application to educational enrollments in states of India. Demography 2001;38(1):115–32.

[12] Ramlagan S, Peltzer K, Phaswana-Mafuya N. Social capital and health among older adults in South Africa. BMC Geriatr 2013;13:100. doi: 10.1186/1471-2318-13-100.

[13] Cohen S, Kamarck T, Mermelstein R. A global measure of perceived stress. J Health Soc Behav 1983;24:385–96. doi: 10.2307/2136404.

[14] Kessler RC, Ustün TB. The World Mental Health (WMH) Survey initiative version of the World Health Organization (WHO) composite international diagnostic interview (CIDI). Int J Methods Psychiatr Res 2004;13(2):93–121.

[15] Vancampfort D, Stubbs B, Koyanagi A. Physical chronic conditions, multimorbidity and sedentary behavior amongst middle-aged and older adults in six low- and middle-income countries. Int J Behav Nutr Phys Act 2017;14(1):147. doi: 10.1186/s12966-017-0602-z.

[16] Peltzer K, Hewlett S, Yawson AE, Moynihan P, Preet R, Wu F, et al. Prevalence of loss of all teeth (edentulism) and associated factors in older adults in China, Ghana,

India, Mexico, Russia and South Africa. Int J Environ Res Public Health 2014;11(11):11308–24. https://doi.org/10.3390/ijerph111111308.

[17] Chobanian AV, Bakris GL, Black HR, Cushman WC, Green LA, Izzo Jr JL, et al. The seventh report of the joint national committee on prevention, detection, evaluation, and treatment of high blood pressure: the JNC 7 report. JAMA 2003;289(19):2560–71.

[18] Arokiasamy P, Uttamacharya, Kowal P, Capistrant BD, Gildner TE, Thiele E, et al. Chronic noncommunicable diseases in 6 low- and middle-income countries: findings from wave 1 of the World Health Organization's Study on Global Ageing and Adult Health (SAGE). Am J Epidemiol 2017;185(6):414-28. doi: 10.1093/aje/kww125.

[19] Ustün T, Kostanjsek N, Chatterji S, Rehm J, eds. Measuring health and disability: manual for WHO Disability Assessment Schedule (WHODAS 2.0). Geneva, Switzerland: WHO, 2010.

[20] Rose GA. The diagnosis of ischaemic heart pain and intermittent claudication in field surveys. Bull World Health Organ 1962;27:645–58.

[21] World Health Organisation. World report on disability. Malta: WHO, 2011.

[22] World Health Organization. Diet, nutrition, and the prevalence of chronic diseases. Geneva, Switzerland: WHO, 2003.

[23] Bull FC, Maslin TS, Armstrong T. Global physical activity questionnaire (GPAQ): nine country reliability and validity study. J Phys Act Health 2009;6(6):790–804.

[24] US Department of Health and Human Services and US Department of Agriculture. 2015- 2020 dietary guidelines for Americans, 2015, appendix alcohol. URL: https://health.gov/our-work/food-nutrition/2015-2020-dietary-guidelines/guidelines/appendix-9/.

[25] World Health Organization. Guidelines for controlling and monitoring the tobacco epidemic. Geneva, Switzerland: WHO, 1998.

[26] Chen Y, Kartsonaki C, Clarke R, Guo Y, Yu C, Bian Z, et al. Characteristics and correlates of sleep duration, daytime napping, snoring and insomnia symptoms among 0.5 million Chinese men and women. Sleep Med 2018;44:67–75. doi:10.1016/j.sleep.2017.11.1131.

[27] Benbir G, Demir AU, Aksu M, Ardic S, Firat H, Itil O, et al. Prevalence of insomnia and its clinical correlates in a general population in Turkey. Psychiatry Clin Neurosci 2015;69(9):543–52. doi:10.1111/pcn.12252.

[28] Sutton DA, Moldofsky H, Badley EM. Insomnia and health problems in Canadians. Sleep 2001;24(6):665–70. doi:10.1093/sleep/24.6.665.

[29] Santos-Silva R, Bittencourt LR, Pires ML, de Mello MT, Taddei JA, Benedito-Silva AA, et al. Increasing trends of sleep complaints in the city of Sao Paulo, Brazil. Sleep Med 2010;11:520–4.

[30] Peltzer K, Pengpid S. Prevalence, social and health correlates of insomnia among persons 15 years and older in Indonesia. Psychol Health Med 2019;24(6):757–68. doi:10.1080/13548506.2019.1566621.

[31] National Institutes of Health State of the Science Conference statement on Manifestations and Management of Chronic Insomnia in Adults, June 13–15, 2005. Sleep 2005;28:1049–57.

[32] Yu C, Shi Z, Lv J, Guo Y, Bian Z, Du H, et al. Dietary Patterns and Insomnia Symptoms in Chinese Adults: The China Kadoorie Biobank. Nutrients 2017;9(3):232. doi:10.3390/nu9030232.

[33] Liu X, Liu L. Sleep habits and insomnia in a sample of elderly persons in China. Sleep 2005;28:1579-87.

SECTION TWO: ACKNOWLEDGMENTS

In: Mexico: Health and Aging
Editors: Supa Pengpid et al.
ISBN: 978-1-53617-950-7

Chapter 17

About the Editors

Supa Pengpid, MPH, DrPH, MBA is a Professor at the ASEAN Institute for Health Development, Mahidol University Thailand since June 2013. She holds a Masterof Sciences in Public Health (MSc), Doctor of Public Health (DrPH in 2001) both from Mahidol University and Master of Business Administration (MBA in 2010) from Regenesys Business School, South Africa. She is a public health expert especially in health behaviour and public health. Her main research interests are health behaviour interventions in areas of chronic diseases prevention, obesity management, alcohol, HIV, TB and sexuality education, gender based violence and health systems research. Email: supaprom@yahoo.com

Karl Peltzer, MA Clin Psych, PhD, Dr Habil is a Research Associate in the Department of Research Administration and Development, University of Limpopo in South Africa. His research focuses on health promotion, risk behaviour and disease prevention, and socio-behavioural interventions on public health subject areas of alcohol, tobacco, cancer, tuberculosis and HIV control, nutrition, physical activity, hypertension, mental health, injury and violence prevention in low- and middle-income countries. Email: kfpeltzer@gmail.com

Joav Merrick, MD, MMedSci, DMSc, born and educated in Denmark is professor of pediatrics, Division of Pediatrics, Hadassah Hebrew University Medical Center, Mt Scopus Campus, Jerusalem, Israel and Kentucky Children's Hospital, University of Kentucky, Lexington, Kentucky United States and professor of public health at the Center for Healthy Development, School of Public Health, Georgia State University, Atlanta, United States, the former medical director of the Health Services, Division for Intellectual and Developmental Disabilities, Ministry of Social Affairs and Social Services, Jerusalem, the founder and director of the National Institute of Child Health and Human Development in Israel. Numerous publications in the field of pediatrics, child health and human development, rehabilitation, intellectual disability, disability, health, welfare, abuse, advocacy, quality of life and prevention. Received the Peter Sabroe Child Award for outstanding work on behalf of Danish Children in 1985 and the International LEGO-Prize ("The Children's Nobel Prize") for an extraordinary contribution towards improvement in child welfare and well-being in 1987. In 2017 appointed a Kentucky Colonel by the Commonwealth of Kentucky, the highest honor the governor can bestow to a person. Email: jmerrick@zahav.net.il

In: Mexico: Health and Aging
Editors: Supa Pengpid et al.
ISBN: 978-1-53617-950-7

Chapter 18

ABOUT THE ASEAN INSTITUTE FOR HEALTH DEVELOPMENT, MAHIDOL UNIVERSITY, SALAYA, PHUTTHAMONTHON, NAKHON PATHOM, THAILAND

The ASEAN Institute for Health Development (AIHD) was established in 1982 as the ASEAN Training Centre for Primary Health Care Development. It was a joint effort of Mahidol University, the Ministry of Public Health and the Department of Technical and Economic Cooperation (DTEC, now TICA) of the Royal Thai Government, with strong support from the Japan International Cooperation Agency (JICA).

AIHD is based on a forward-looking and conceptually challenging perspective on human resource development which aims to support the global strategy of "Health for all" through the primary health care approach advocated by the World Health Organization, an approach which is valid not only for Thailand but also other ASEAN countries.

AIHD has three key missions, namely education and training, technical services, and research and development, focusing on participatory community-based health and related program management, with a special emphasis on facilitating the paradigm shift from a "service-oriented" approach to a "development" approach in order to promote "Health for all" through human capacity building and community empowerment.

Vision

Center of excellence in research, education, professional services for innovative of sustainable health by 2020.

Mission

Provide transformative education for graduates to become leaders in health system management and sustainability. Enhance capacity related of public health workforce in relate to sustainable health development and develop innovative research for sustainable health.

Strategies

Excellence in research for health development models and sustainability. Transformative education. Innovative professional service for sustainable health and wxcellence in management for sustainable organization.

Website

www.aihd.mahidol.ac.th

In: Mexico: Health and Aging
Editors: Supa Pengpid et al.
ISBN: 978-1-53617-950-7

Chapter 19

About the Department of Research Administration and Development, University of Limpopo, Turfloop, South Africa

The Department of Research Administration and Development is a key Department at the University of Limpopo overseeing research performance across the university, developing and implementing policies aligned to the university's strategic plan (UL 2019 - 2023) goal 5, which is improving the university's research standing and status. The department further intends to accelerate professional, quality, efficient research output with the hope to generate funds for the university. Among its key research responsibilities, the department is responsible for managing and directing all aspects of planning, policy, performance, operational support for research and innovation activities and to implement technology transfer and intellectual property (IP) management strategy.

In: Mexico: Health and Aging
Editors: Supa Pengpid et al.
ISBN: 978-1-53617-950-7

Chapter 20

About the National Institute of Child Health and Human Development in Israel

The National Institute of Child Health and Human Development (NICHD) in Israel was established in 1998 as a virtual institute under the auspices of the Medical Director, Ministry of Social Affairs and Social Services in order to function as the research arm for the Office of the Medical Director. In 1998 the National Council for Child Health and Pediatrics, Ministry of Health and in 1999 the Director General and Deputy Director General of the Ministry of Health endorsed the establishment of the NICHD.

Mission

The mission of a National Institute for Child Health and Human Development in Israel is to provide an academic focal point for the scholarly interdisciplinary study of child life, health, public health, welfare, disability, rehabilitation, intellectual disability and related aspects of human development. This mission includes research, teaching, clinical work, information and public service activities in the field of child health and human development.

Service and academic activities

Over the years many activities became focused in the south of Israel due to collaboration with various professionals at the Faculty of Health Sciences (FOHS) at the Ben Gurion University of the Negev (BGU). Since 2000 an affiliation with the Zusman Child Development Center at the Pediatric Division of Soroka University Medical Center has resulted in collaboration around the establishment of the Down Syndrome Clinic at that center. In 2002 a full course on "Disability" was established at the Recanati School for Allied Professions in the Community, FOHS, BGU and in 2005 collaboration was started with the Primary Care Unit of the faculty and disability became part of the master of public health course on "Children and society". In the academic year 2005-2006 a one semester course on "Aging with disability" was started as part of the master of science program in gerontology in our collaboration with the Center for Multidisciplinary Research in Aging. In 2010 collaborations with the Division of Pediatrics, Hadassah Hebrew University Medical Center, Jerusalem, Israel around the National Down Syndrome Center and teaching students and residents about intellectual and developmental disabilities as part of their training at this campus.

Research activities

The affiliated staff have over the years published work from projects and research activities in this national and international collaboration. In the year 2000 the International Journal of Adolescent Medicine and Health and in 2005 the International Journal on Disability and Human Development of De Gruyter Publishing House (Berlin and New York) were affiliated with the National Institute of Child Health and Human Development. From

2008 also the International Journal of Child Health and Human Development (Nova Science, New York), the International Journal of Child and Adolescent Health (Nova Science) and the Journal of Pain Management (Nova Science) affiliated and from 2009 the International Public Health Journal (Nova Science) and Journal of Alternative Medicine Research (Nova Science). All peer-reviewed international journals.

National collaborations

Nationally the NICHD works in collaboration with the Faculty of Health Sciences, Ben Gurion University of the Negev; Department of Physical Therapy, Sackler School of Medicine, Tel Aviv University; Autism Center, Assaf HaRofeh Medical Center; National Rett and PKU Centers at Chaim Sheba Medical Center, Tel HaShomer; Department of Physiotherapy, Haifa University; Department of Education, Bar Ilan University, Ramat Gan, Faculty of Social Sciences and Health Sciences; College of Judea and Samaria in Ariel and in 2011 affiliation with Center for Pediatric Chronic Diseases and National Center for Down Syndrome, Department of Pediatrics, Hadassah Hebrew University Medical Center, Mount Scopus Campus, Jerusalem.

International collaborations

Internationally with the Department of Disability and Human Development, College of Applied Health Sciences, University of Illinois at Chicago; Strong Center for Developmental Disabilities, Golisano Children's Hospital at Strong, University of Rochester School of Medicine and Dentistry, New York; Centre on Intellectual Disabilities, University of Albany, New York; Centre for Chronic Disease Prevention and Control, Health Canada, Ottawa; Chandler Medical Center and Children's Hospital, Kentucky Children's Hospital, Section of Adolescent Medicine, University of Kentucky, Lexington; Chronic Disease Prevention and Control Research

Center, Baylor College of Medicine, Houston, Texas; Division of Neuroscience, Department of Psychiatry, Columbia University, New York; Institute for the Study of Disadvantage and Disability, Atlanta; Center for Autism and Related Disorders, Department Psychiatry, Children's Hospital Boston, Boston; Department of Pediatric and Adolescent Medicine, Western Michigan University Homer Stryker MD School of Medicine, Kalamazoo, Michigan, United States; Department of Paediatrics, Child Health and Adolescent Medicine, Children's Hospital at Westmead, Westmead, Australia; International Centre for the Study of Occupational and Mental Health, Düsseldorf, Germany; Centre for Advanced Studies in Nursing, Department of General Practice and Primary Care, University of Aberdeen, Aberdeen, United Kingdom; Quality of Life Research Center, Copenhagen, Denmark; Nordic School of Public Health, Gottenburg, Sweden, Scandinavian Institute of Quality of Working Life, Oslo, Norway; The Department of Applied Social Sciences (APSS) of The Hong Kong Polytechnic University Hong Kong.

Targets

Our focus is on research, international collaborations, clinical work, teaching and policy in health, disability and human development and to establish the NICHD as a permanent institute in Israel.

Contact

Professor Joav Merrick, MD, MMedSci, DMSc
National Institute of Child Health and Human Development,
Jerusalem, Israel.
Email: jmerrick@zahav.net.il

SECTION THREE: INDEX

INDEX

A

B

C

D

E

F

G

H

I

J

K

L

M

N

O

P

Q

R

S

T

U

V

W

X